ENDORSEMENTS

"This story will shake you to the core, it will anger, enlighten, inspire, give you hope, and make you giggle. Mostly it will convince you that without the shadow of a doubt, cancer can be cured, and that the monster behind the curtain does not even exist."

Alex Lubarsky, author of *The Art of Selling The Art of Healing:*
How the Rebels of Today are Creating the Health Care of Tomorrow;
and Why your Life Depends on It

"This book is such a fascinating combination of personal story and details on the suppression of holistic cancer (and other disease) therapies. Beljanski took up the challenge of presenting her brilliant father's research and ideas in a world dominated by conventional approaches. As an Advocate for people with cancer, and a survivor who chose other paths than conventional, I can appreciate the effort it took to bring ideas forward that are resented and repressed. This knowledge is critical to our ability to make informed treatment decisions."

Ann E. Fonfa, President of Annie Appleseed Project

"Sylvie's book is a true winner. She discusses a groundbreaking scientific approach to understanding and treating cancer based on her father's solid scientific findings while also portraying her personal trials and tribulations in trying to continue her father's research and clinical work. All of this is presented while showing how the medical and scientific establishment go to almost any length to try to stop innovation and treatment with natural unpatentable remedies, so that the pharmaceutically driven status quo can be maintained."

Michael B. Schachter, MD, CNS, Director of the
Schachter Center for Complementary Medicine

T0163628

"*Winning the War on Cancer: An Epic Journey Towards a Natural Cure* goes beyond the usual low-toxin advice to share beating and preventing cancer at the DNA level based on the research of scientist Mirko Beljanski. Sylvie Beljanski, his daughter, questions why his nontoxic, scientifically validated protocols for cancer were once rejected by the medical community but over time have now come to be recognized for their efficacy and benefits; she shares where to find the plant-and nucleic acid-based protocols that are effective at saving lives."

David Steinman, author *Diet for a Poisoned Planet* and
*Safe Trip to Eden: 10 Steps to Save Planet Earth from the
Global Warming Meltdown,* publisher of *Healthy Living Magazine*

"Sylvie Beljanski writes a 'must-read' if you are involved in any way with cancer and chronic disease. Whether a current patient or caregiver, a survivor, a researcher, an author/speaker, or a physician, the information in this book is ground-breaking, exciting, and essential to know. Indeed, even if you do not have anything to do with cancer and chronic disease currently, with the new data leaning towards 1 in 2 people receiving a cancer diagnosis in their lifetimes, you will want to read this book! The book is easy to read, as told through Sylvie's viewpoint as first a child and then as an adult professional seeking truth and justice in the medical and scientific field. Filled with excellent scientific information and sources, it is also an educational journey. It was so sincere, captivating, poignant, and educational—all at the same time: I loved it!"

Annie Brandt, Survivor/Thriver,
Founder and President Emerita of Best Answer for Cancer Foundation.

"With *Winning the War on Cancer: The Epic Journey Towards a Natural Cure*, Sylvie Beljanski offers an eye-opening glimpse into natural cancer cures, and the many lives they've saved and changed. It's a powerful journey of dedication and discovery, changing the face of cancer research, and offering real hope to the millions of cancer patients struggling to survive."

Michele Cagan, Editor, *Health Sciences Institute Members Alert*

"Throughout history, those brilliant individuals who have threatened the egos and reputations of the establishment, and/or the profits of industries, have been ridiculed, persecuted, or prosecuted. This is particularly so in the science and health industries. When I had pondered this myopic situation, Albert Einstein came to mind, and now, Beljanski."

David P. Michaels, President, Foreign Press Association (FPA-USA)

"The heroine of this story is a lawyer who through a series of adventures has dedicated her life to show the world her father's important life-extending products. This quest has resulted in life-threatening adventures, run-ins with some pretty shady characters, and a validation of her father's scientific research."

James Grutsch PhD, Adjunct Assistant Professor of Epidemiology, University of Illinois at Chicago; Chief Analytics Officer, Rhythmalytics, LLC.

WINNING
THE WAR ON
CANCER

The Epic Journey Towards a **Natural Cure**

SYLVIE BELJANSKI

NEW YORK

LONDON • NASHVILLE • MELBOURNE • VANCOUVER

WINNING THE WAR ON CANCER

Published in New York, New York, by Morgan James Publishing. Morgan James is a trademark of Morgan James, LLC.
www.MorganJamesPublishing.com

The Morgan James Speakers Group can bring authors to your live event. For more information or to book an event visit The Morgan James Speakers Group at www.TheMorganJamesSpeakersGroup.com.

ISBN 978-1-68350-724-6 paperback
ISBN 978-1-68350-725-3 hardcover
ISBN 978-1-68350-726-0 eBook
Library of Congress Control Number: 2017912848

Cover Designs by:
Chris Treccani @ 3 Dog Creative
Glenn Zagoren @ Zagoren Collective

Interior Design by:
Megan Whitney Dillon
Creative Ninja Designs
megan@creativeninjadesigns.com

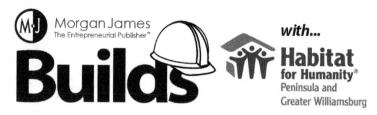

In an effort to support local communities, raise awareness and funds, Morgan James Publishing donates a percentage of all book sales for the life of each book to Habitat for Humanity Peninsula and Greater Williamsburg.

Get involved today! Visit
www.MorganJamesBuilds.com

DISCLAIMER

The information provided in this book is designed to provide helpful support on the subject discussed. This book is not meant to be used, nor should be used, to diagnose or treat any medical condition. Products, services, information, and other content are provided for informational purposes only and are not meant to be used, nor should be used, to diagnose or treat any medical condition. The publisher and the author make no legal or medical claims, and they are not engaged in rendering medical, legal or other professional advice or services. Please consult a physician or other healthcare professional regarding any medical or health related diagnosis and treatment options.

This book is a work of non-fiction. However, some names have been altered to protect people's privacy and some events have been condensed for the sake of the story. This memoir certainly represents the author's story based on her own point of view, but, given the limitations of perception and memory, makes no claim to objective certainty.

To Mamée, my grandmother, who gave me the tools
to ride this journey and to write about it.

And

To all those whose words of support, kindness, and
wisdom will continue to echo in me.

Thank you.

CONTENTS

FOREWORD

I first learned of Sylvie Beljanski's work, and the work of her father Mirko Beljanski, PhD, when the Beljanski Foundation reached out to the Alliance for Natural Health USA, where I have served as the executive director for almost ten years. We were lobbying at the time to pass legislation that would have made it legal to share information about the health benefits of natural foods and dietary supplements when that information is supported by peer reviewed, scientific studies. Sylvie was interested in supporting our efforts, because she shares my concern that the public cannot legally learn about the empirically proven benefits of natural remedies. Unfortunately, this limited access to natural healing options isn't the exception to the rule. Generally the laws are stacked against those who wish to use natural medicine to maintain optimal health.

Having worked on Capitol Hill for more than a dozen years, I have seen things that make me wish, at times, for blissful ignorance. The stories about "horse trading"—Congressional support for legislation in exchange for reciprocal concessions, rather than to further the public interest—are true. Many of our laws aren't designed for your benefit or mine. Rather, they are architected by the companies and special interests who desire more control over the regulatory environment that impacts their bottom line. This happens in all sectors, but my area of expertise is in nature, which doesn't play by industry's rules.

Think about it. We don't own nature. For example, no one owns all of the aloe vera plants. Anyone can grow aloe vera, and anyone can sell the aloe vera that they have grown. You and I can use that aloe vera to soothe sunburns or calm an upset stomach. By law, Mother Nature and her bountiful natural remedies cannot be patented. Period. Sure, recipes and delivery systems that are invented can be patented, and therefore owned, by the inventor. But for the most part, if it's natural, it cannot be owned by one, because it already belongs to us all.

Now, pharmaceutical companies love synthetic medicines that they can patent, because synthetic ingredients are cheap to manufacture, and not only do the companies enjoy sole ownership, but the Food and Drug Administration (FDA), which regulates drugs, guarantees market exclusivity of these new, patented drugs for a period of five and a half years. This means no other drugs can be marketed if they would impact sales, but this doesn't apply to natural remedies that are already being legally sold. What pharmaceutical companies don't love is competition from natural medicines they cannot control or own, which can oftentimes work better than their synthetic drugs and without the nasty side effects. So what do you think these companies might do in turn? That's right, they lobby members of Congress.

They lobby to eliminate our ability to make meaningful choices about our own health and well-being by removing information, as well as the natural alternatives to pharmaceutical drugs themselves, from the marketplace. Surprisingly, it really is illegal for a supplement company, for example, to list the specific health benefits of their products on the label. They can provide general information about how nutrients affect the structure or function of the body, but they can't tell you that cinnamon and bitter melon, for example, lower blood sugar. Why not, when countless diabetics would benefit from this information? It doesn't make sense until you realize that, because it's not a patented drug, it's much, much less expensive. And if everyone knew there was an affordable, natural alterative to diabetes drugs, well, that market exclusivity would be meaningless as those wishing for a safer alternative would flock towards cinnamon, bitter melon, and the countless other safer options to diabetes drugs.

Drug companies don't just want to block the information we get about natural medicines; they want these products off of store shelves altogether. The end game for them is a preapproval system, where supplements have to go through the same steps that drugs do to get approved. Simply put, this would cost hundreds of millions of dollars for natural substances that, because they can't be patented, don't enjoy the same market protections synthetic drugs do. Dozens of companies make cinnamon supplements. How could any one of them afford to spend hundreds of millions of dollars for studies when they won't recoup that investment on the other end? They can't, and therefore such a requirement would be the end of these products. And drug companies know this.

Nevertheless, there is concern that drugs may be a safer bet. But is this really true?

The FDA regulates both drugs and dietary supplements, including herbs like Beljanski's *Pao pereira* and the *Rauwolfia vomitoria* extract. In fact, the FDA tracks adverse health events that are reported from consumers and patients who believe they were injured from taking both drugs and dietary supplements. In 2016, there were 8,536 dietary supplement adverse events reported to the FDA's Center for Food Safety and Applied Nutrition's Adverse Event Reporting System. That same year, there were 1,184,764 drug-related adverse events reported to the FDA.

Then there is the common sense test. Cinnamon is a food. I know dozens of integrative physicians who recommend it to their patients, because they have seen the benefits. In fact, a lot of this comes down to common sense.

I, like many people, found my way into the natural health world because of my own health struggles. I didn't have cancer or AIDs. I had Hashimoto's, an autoimmune thyroid disease, and profound endocrine and gastrointestinal dysfunction that destroyed my ability to function normally at age thirty-one. After delivering my daughter, my body shut down in many ways, leaving me severely depressed, fatigued, and unable to digest the food I ate. I saw dozens of doctors who told me I should just take prescription drugs for the rest of my life and there was nothing more they could do for me. I was told my condition was irreversible. But instead of giving up, I became my own advocate and learned everything there was to know about my health problems. I read over one hundred books, attended alternative and complementary medical seminars, and started seeing integrative physicians who use both allopathic and alternative, natural approaches to medicine. It took several years, and it was the hardest thing I have ever done, but using foods and dietary supplements, I'm much, much better. I no longer have Hashimoto's, and I function at about 90 percent on most days.

My common sense questions are: "Why did none of the initial doctors I saw— the ones my insurance company worked with—know how to help me?" and "Why did I literally have to go to medical seminars and go completely 'outside' of the medical system as we know it, to learn about the natural foods and supplements I needed to heal?" Twenty-seven million people in America have thyroid disease.

90 percent of them have Hashimoto's, the autoimmune disease I had. "How many of these people are struggling to get through the day, when they don't have to, because their doctors also told them there was nothing more to be done to help them?" My last question is, "Why in the world, when over half of all Americans are chronically ill and more than one in three will have cancer at some point in our lives, are we allowing our public and elected officials to work with pharmaceutical companies to limit access to the medicines that can actually reverse disease and restore wellbeing?"

The brilliant Mirko Beljanski, PhD, found miracles in nature—*Pao pereira*, a tree native to the Amazon, and *Rauwolfia vomitoria*, which is extracted from an African root bark—that proved to heal countless patients from cancer and AIDS. You would think these would be household names, and we would all be celebrating this major milestone in the war on cancer. But we aren't. In fact, most people don't know anything about these two natural remedies. "WHY?" Sylvie Beljanski tells us in the pages that follow. Beljanski's story is critical, not just for those with cancer and AIDS, but for all of us, because either we, or our family members, now or in the future, need natural medicine to thrive. It belongs to us. And if we don't ask the questions, and if we don't fight for truth as Sylvie Beljanski did, we may find ourselves suffering needlessly, both from the chronic illnesses that are ravaging this country, and the deadly medicines that are used to treat them.

Gretchen DuBeau, Esq.

Executive Director

Alliance for Natural Health, USA

INTRODUCTION

T he "War on Cancer" was declared on December 23, 1971. On that day, President Richard Nixon signed into law the National Cancer Act, which allocated $1.5 billion for cancer research over the course of three years. Although the legislation never mentioned the word "war," Nixon declared: "The same kind of concentrated effort that split the atom and took man to the moon should be turned toward conquering this dread disease."

So, how have we done?

In 2011, on the fortieth anniversary of the National Cancer Act, Dr. Otis Brawley delivered the following assessment on CNN: "The war is still being waged, and much of the optimism has faded. This year, more than 500,000 Americans will die of cancer. Obviously, this is a war not won, and it is appropriate to ask: What have we gotten from this forty-year war?"[1]

The latest World Cancer Report, released in 2014 by the World Health Organization on World Cancer Day, predicted new cancer cases will rise from an estimated 14 million annually in 2012 to 22 million within two decades. Over the same period, cancer deaths are predicted to rise from 8.2 million a year to 13 million.[2]

Certainly, progress has been made in some areas, and there are some success stories. But often, those can be linked to legislation and financial resources devoted to early detection, rather than improvement of the treatments themselves. For example, in the US, the rate of new lung cancer cases has steadily declined as fewer people smoke. The decrease of new colon cancer cases has been attributed in part to more people getting colonoscopies, which

1

can prevent cancer through the removal of pre-cancerous polyps. As for the decline in the number of reported prostate cancer cases, it is mainly due to the fact that fewer cases are now being detected: PSA testing (blood test used primarily to screen for prostate cancer) is no longer being routinely used because of high rates of over-diagnosis, according to the American Cancer Society.[3]

Other cancers are on the rise, including leukemia, cancers of the tongue, tonsil, small intestine, liver, pancreas, kidney, thyroid, vulvar, pancreas, as well as endometrial cancers, male breast cancers, testicular cancers, and throat cancers.[3]

Some researchers are looking at numbers, scrambling for explanations and silver linings. They suggest that since we have an aging population, the cancer rate increases, but if you adjust for the aging of America, the cancer rate is actually declining.

The fact is that at the beginning of the last century, one person in twenty would get cancer. In the 1940s it was one out of every sixteen individuals. In the 1970s it was one person out of ten. Today, one out of three individuals will get cancer in the course of their lives. Sadly, even the incidence of childhood cancer follows the same trend, averaging a 0.6 percent increase per year since the mid-1970s and resulting in an overall increase of 24 percent over the last forty years.[4]

Money is not the real problem. Cancer is an industry worth billions. As Dr. Margaret Cuomo (sister of New York Governor Andrew Cuomo) wrote in 2013: "More than 40 years after the war on cancer was declared, we have spent billions fighting the good fight. The National Cancer Institute has spent some $90 billion on research and treatment during that time. Some 260 nonprofit organizations in the United States have dedicated themselves to cancer—more than the number established for heart disease, AIDS, Alzheimer's disease, and stroke combined. Together, these 260 organizations have budgets that top $2.2 billion."[5]

In 2014 the National Cancer Institute (NCI) stated that the medical costs of cancer care were $125 billion, with a projected 39 percent increase to $173 billion by 2020.

Working with the self-fulfilling assumption that the cancer market will grow, not shrink, the cancer industry has lost its way. "The search for knowledge has become an end unto itself rather than the means to an end," explained Clifton Leaf, author of an article entitled "Why we are losing the war on cancer?" that made the cover of *Fortune* magazine in 2004.[6]

No doubt that money has bought us a tremendous amount of knowledge: "Scientific discovery has given us a golden toolbox of genome sequencing and artificial intelligence programs that can characterize individual patient cancers rather than broad groups," wrote health journalist Danny Buckland.[7]

However, that knowledge, more often than not, has not translated into real improvement of cancer outcomes. Survival gains for the most common forms of cancer are still measured in additional *months* of life, not years.[6]

Meanwhile, the cost of cancer drugs has skyrocketed in the last fifteen years. The average cancer drug price for approximately one year of therapy was less than $10,000 before 2000. By 2005, it had increased from $30,000 to $50,000. In 2012, twelve of the thirteen new drugs approved for cancer indications were priced above $100,000 per year of therapy.[8] With typical out-of-pocket expenses at 20 to 30 percent, many patients (estimated 10 to 20 percent) are priced out and may decide not to take the treatment, or may compromise significantly on the treatment plan.[9]

The public is craving natural solutions that are effective yet affordable. Nearly half of patients with cancer reported that they started taking dietary supplements after being given a diagnosis of cancer[10] and 58 percent of individuals who consume dietary supplements report they do so for the prevention or treatment of cancer.[11]

Every day oncologists are challenged to provide advice to patients about which supplements are safe and effective to use to treat cancer or the side effects of cancer therapy, and which supplements are antagonistic to standard treatment with chemotherapy, radiation, and/or immunotherapy. And they find it difficult to answer, even though research is routinely conducted with natural products.

More than a thousand clinical trials of dietary supplements are reported on ClinicalTrials.gov, yet the FDA has not approved any food or dietary supplement to prevent cancer, halt its growth, or prevent its recurrence. The successful use of many extracts from plants collected for their potential medical application contrasts sharply with the failure of clinical trials to lead to the regulatory approval of common foods and dietary supplements (such as green tea, pomegranate, lycopene, soy, mistletoe, vitamins C, D, and E, selenium, resveratrol) as treatments for cancer.[12]

Clinical trials of plant extracts may be conducted either by a dietary supplement manufacturer, or by a drug company. Some dietary supplement manufacturers may want to validate the safety and efficacy that is claimed for a traditional herbal medicine. But without patent protection, the dietary supplement manufacturer faces price pressure from competitors and cannot obtain enough profits from high product prices to pay for the costs of large clinical trials. The manufacturer will have to rely on small studies that will never lead to FDA approval. On the other hand, many drug companies may want to test the clinical activity of a purified or semi-purified compound derived from some plant extract, that they will then have to modify and synthesize before seeking patent protection. Those trials are not aimed at obtaining FDA approval for a natural substance, but are part of the early process of drug development. Natural products have long been recognized as excellent leads for drug development: the earliest anticancer drugs approved by the FDA and derived from natural products were the vinca alkaloids (vincristine in 1963 and vinblastine in 1965), which were isolated from Madagascar periwinkle plants found growing in Jamaica and the Philippines.[13] Similarly, Paclitaxel was first isolated from the bark of the Pacific yew tree (*Taxus brevifolia*) in the state of Washington as part of a collection program undertaken by the U.S. Department of Agriculture on behalf of the National Cancer Institute.[14]

Unfortunately, when a molecule is modified and synthesized in order to conform to patent law requirements, it often becomes highly toxic. However, since it is the only one able to command a substantial return on investment, it will be the only one considered for development.

In the end, very few natural compounds are seriously researched.

In 1951, my father, Mirko Beljanski, PhD, a biologist-biochemist, joined the famous Pasteur Institute in Paris, France. Convinced that there was value in a different approach to cancer, he started to entirely rethink the origin of the disease. As he tested his revolutionary theory, he went on to develop natural molecules able to selectively block cancerous cell multiplication without killing healthy cells. When he began to accumulate scientific evidence and publish his results, he ran into major opposition. The conventional oncology community ostracized him, despite the fact that his theories on cancer treatment were aimed at complementing chemotherapy and radiation, not replacing them. That did not prevent François Mitterrand in 1992, then President of France, to turn to Beljanski's plant extracts during his battle with advanced prostate cancer. What happened next started off my own journey.

I would not have survived this epic adventure without the selfless support of the many people I met along the way. Thanks to their support in the past two decades, The Beljanski Foundation has grown into a registered nonprofit organization whose mission is to further Dr. Beljanski's research within a network of high-profile research institutions around the world.

This legacy is so important, yet so fragile. My intent for *Winning the War On Cancer: The Epic Journey Towards a Natural Cure* is to deliver a story and share this wealth of knowledge while I still can.

CHAPTER ONE
FINDING MY VOICE

"You were born with the ability to change someone's life—
don't ever waste it."

DALE PARTRIDGE

I have the privilege of educating the public about cancer and the research program pursued by The Beljanski Foundation.*

My message is a positive one, backed by real science, serious studies, and published data. A jaw-dropping cancer research program is ongoing in the U.S., yet it remains little known. In the face of the rising occurrence rates of different cancers, the results of this research could save many lives. That knowledge makes me relentless in reaching beyond the status quo, and insisting on sharing this groundbreaking science. Every new publication brings me sheer joy.

After all, that's what my life is all about now.

Just a few months ago, I had the opportunity to give a presentation at NAVEL Expo–a Long Island wellness event. My good friend, Alex Lubarsky, Founder and CEO of Health Media Group and organizer of the event, booked me as a keynote speaker. I was extremely eager to deliver my presentation and share the quality and originality of the latest results from

---

* www.beljanski.org

The Beljanski Foundation's sponsored research concerning cancer stem cells. As I was the speaker of the hour, I looked forward to having the undivided attention of all the attendees at the trade show.

Cancer stem cells* are crucial to cancer research because they are those cells known to be resistant to chemotherapy. They also induce relapse and metastasis (when cancer travels from one part of the body to another) by giving rise to new tumors.

Over the past sixty years, cancer death rates in the U.S. have decreased only slightly. Those years have also seen billions of dollars invested in research that have turned cancer into a multi trillion-dollar industry. Traditional treatments for cancer include surgery, chemotherapy, and radiation. But even though these treatments can shrink or eliminate tumors, often, the cancer can return with a vengeance. This is due to the cancer stem cells.

According to research, cancer cells are not all created equal. A malignant tumor or the circulating cancerous cells of leukemia, for instance, can harbor many different cell types. The stem cell theory of cancer proposes that among all cancerous cells, only a few act as stem cells.

The concept that cancer is primarily driven by a minute population of stem cells has important implications. As the Ludwig Center for Cancer Stem Cell Research and Medicine explains:

> "Many new anticancer therapies are evaluated based on their ability to shrink tumors, but if the therapies are not killing the cancer stem cells, the tumor will soon grow back (often with a vexing resistance to the previously used therapy). An analogy would be a weeding technique that is evaluated based on how low it can chop the weed stalks—but no matter how low the weeds are cut, if the roots aren't taken out, the weeds will just grow back. Another important implication is that it is the cancer stem cells that give rise to metastases and can also act as a reservoir of cancer

---

*   A stem cell is an unspecialized cell that can divide and replace its own numbers indefinitely and also give rise to cells that have the potential to differentiate into one or more specific cell types. What starts out as an unspecialized, no-name cell may turn into a brain cell, or a muscle cell or a blood cell. This unique power of stem cells to divide and differentiate accounts for the whole process of our normal growth and development. However, cancers can hijack this power leading to cancer stem cells that promote tumor growth and metastasis, as they continue to multiply, and have the ability to produce a variety of cancer cell types.

cells that may cause a relapse after surgery, radiation, or chemotherapy has eliminated all observable signs of a cancer."[1]

Given the importance of this topic, you can imagine how excited I was to present one of the latest studies that was done through The Beljanski Foundation's research program in collaboration with University of Kansas Medical Center (KUMC). Research has shown that both plant extracts developed by my late father, Mirko Beljanski, namely the *Pao pereira* extract and the *Rauwolfia vomitoria* extract, worked beautifully against pancreatic cancer stem cells, as well as ovarian cancer stem cells. Pancreatic and ovarian cancers are very difficult to treat because they are usually diagnosed very late, and the tumor cells generally become resistant to the drugs chosen for treatment. However, in the previously stated experiment, all the cancer stems cells were completely eradicated by natural extracts, which are not toxic to healthy cells, and in only a matter of hours!

My presentation had been highly publicized, and my picture was even on the cover of the NAVEL Expo magazine. I knew the data I held in my possession was nothing less than stunning. Very excited, and only a little nervous, I walked into the room already filled beyond capacity with hundreds of people waiting to hear what I had to say.

I took out my USB drive to place it in the computer and suddenly realized in horror that there was no computer. In fact, there was no projector either! How was I going to present my data?

I swallowed hard and tried to compose myself, but my heart was beating so loud I was sure it could be heard by even those standing in the back. Without a word to my waiting audience, I raced out of the room in a panic to find Alex and beg his help.

"Please Alex! My presentation is NOW and I have no computer and I have no projector and the people are waiting and I..."

I don't even know if I finished my sentence. I had to get back to the room pronto and say something to all those people waiting to hear about cancer research. Despite my high heels, I literally sprinted back to the room, and took a deep breath.

Usually my presentations were data-driven, meaning I carefully avoided making it personal. I did not feel comfortable with anything personal. Ever. I felt that since I did not have the proper scientific background or credentials, I was not entitled to a voice or opinion. I was thinking of myself as an anonymous vector presenting data on behalf of The Beljanski Foundation. Sure the Foundation was my creation, the meting out of my promise to my father to carry on his work, and it was my idea to pursue this avenue of research with KUMC, but still I felt that it was not my research, my data.

However, we were waiting for the equipment, so I had no choice but to improvise. I could not just stare back at people who were staring at me, still waiting to hear about cancer research. I had to start somewhere.

"How many of you have heard my presentations before?"

Very few raised their hand, so I felt I needed to introduce myself. I started with the obvious—my French accent—which always made me feel intimidated about public speaking. To me, it was the elephant in the room.

"Do you have any idea why a French lady would come on this beautiful Sunday afternoon to Long Island to speak to you about cancer when I am not a cancer survivor and I am not a cancer researcher?"

And there it was. Nothing in my background had prepared me to be there on that stage one day. It is even fair to say that growing up I wasn't really interested in science. My focus was entirely different. In fact, I eventually passed the Paris (France) bar exam, and was then invited to join a New York law firm. So you see how far off I was from being a science scholar.

My parents were both scientists working at the Pasteur Institute in Paris. My mother, Monique, was a research engineer and my father, Mirko Beljanski, a Director of Research with a PhD in molecular biology (having received his degree in 1951 from the Sorbonne in Paris). They worked together for forty-nine years. It was my father who discovered the anticancer use and anti-viral benefits of the specific botanical extracts which were the topic of my presentation. As a self-acknowledged workaholic passionate about biology, he published and left a body of 133 peer-reviewed publications.*

---

*   See Appendix 1: Scientific Publications of Mirko Beljanski

A number of these publications were read by a group of French doctors who became very interested in working with my father to develop plant extracts and distribute them to patients. When I was growing up, there was an ongoing line of people coming to the apartment crying because they had been diagnosed with cancer. As a little girl I thought, "Good, we're getting rid of them," when they left. But inevitably three or four months later, they were coming back with flowers saying they were doing better. It seemed endless—this array of people showing up crying, then returning with gifts, chocolate, and flowers—because they were doing better. Growing up, I felt

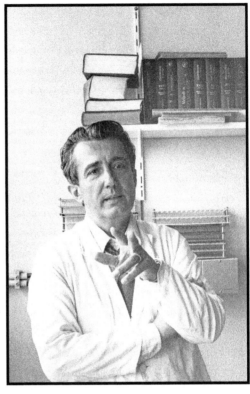

Dr. Mirko Beljanski circa 1972 (Photograph: Monique Beljanski - © The Beljanski Foundation, Inc.)

my life was absolutely overrun by those people, and I swore I would never get involved in that...

It was another lonely, miserable day. The sun was beaming through the large kitchen windows of our Paris apartment, but I felt cold. Cold and lonely. I fiddled with the bowl of lentil soup that had grown just as cold as I felt while I had been sitting at the table trying to eat. I wasn't hungry. My parents had, once again, left me to finish lunch alone and I felt tossed out of their lives ... once again. What was so important about plant extracts, anyway? Why did they always have to be at that laboratory day and night and couldn't seem to find the time to listen to what I had to say or understand how I felt about anything? And even when they were home, we were constantly invaded by some sick-looking men and women looking for help and handouts.

I felt the tears roll down my face and watched as they dropped and disappeared, one by one, into the bowl of soup like tiny ice crystals tumbling from the sky to dance on a lonely skating rink. It was bad enough that those people were coming to the apartment all hours of the night. In the morning, it was the same thing. The tall, thin woman that got us all out of bed was particularly frightening. Although she wore a bright red beret with a large, multi-colored feather sticking out of the top, I knew she was bald. Why did my parents want to help another ghastly woman? And what about me? Didn't they know I was sick too?

By all standards, I was a well-fed, well-clothed, well-schooled little girl; but I was craving for attention, and confusing attention with love. I remember thinking: "If only I was bacteria, or something like that, maybe they would pay attention to me."

———————

Little did I know, as I was growing up, that the two extraordinary plant products my father discovered and perfected would have such astoundingly far-reaching effects. They changed my parents' lives and they changed the history of France. They eventually changed my own life in ways I could have never imagined.

In 1990 French President François Mitterrand was officially diagnosed with advanced prostate cancer. He was two years into his second seven-year term of office at the time. Actually, he had been sick for several years already, but the French President's health situation had been kept secret for as long as possible. By 1992, with three years left in his second term, the President was very obviously sick and surgery could not be delayed any further.

After surgery, the President's surgeon declared that nothing could be done as the cancer had already spread too far. He suggested administering morphine for the pain, and preparing the country for early elections.

But Mitterrand—as any good French story goes—had a mistress, and his mistress's great family doctor was known to have outstanding results with prostate cancer by using my father's products. Dr. Philip de Kuyper, who had a thriving practice in the city of Versailles, was immediately invited to come to the Elysée Palace (the French equivalent of the White House), and see if he could help Mitterrand.

Dr. de Kuyper was quick to oblige. When he arrived at the Elysée Palace, Mitterrand was lying in his bed.

"What can you do for me? Help me suffer less? Help me die peacefully?"

"I think we can do better than that Mr. President. Based on my experience and if you are serious about taking the pills I am going to prescribe you, I think we can not only slow down the progression of the disease, but we can reasonably hope to get you back on your feet."

"Nothing would be more important to me than to finish my work."

So, Mitterrand began taking the *Pao pereira* and the *Rauwolfia vomitoria* extracts. Against all odds, he started to get better.

Of course, at the same time, there were government ministers who had heard from the official surgeon that it was time to prepare the country for early elections. On one hand, there were officials scrambling to prepare a funeral and early elections—with politicians positioning themselves to take over. On the other hand, the President was improving with each passing day and becoming less willing to let go of power. A tense situation arose between these officials who were ready and willing to seize power, and a President who was not ready, nor willing, to relinquish that power.

The President was thankful for the life-saving extracts. Despite the fact that all the traditional doctors and protégés of the Elysée Palace were raging an open war against Dr. de Kuyper, describing this—until then—well-respected physician as a quack practicing quackery.[2] In 1995, in an interview published in *Paris Match* (a prestigious French news magazine) Mitterrand acknowledged that the products Dr. de Kuyper was giving him were truly making a difference in his health.[3]

In May 1995, Mitterrand, against all odds, was able to finish his second term and leave the Elysée Palace with all the honors and respect of a living president. A few months after leaving office, he decided that it was time to stop all medications, and let nature take its course. Reportedly on January 6, 1996 Mitterrand, a long-time opponent of euthanasia, was given a fatal intravenous injection to end his suffering, at his own request.[4]

As long as Mitterrand was alive, nothing happened. My father was protected.

However, shortly after Mitterrand passed away, the officials who had been greatly disturbed with Mitterrand's unexpected recovery came back for revenge against my father and Dr. de Kuyper. The idea that integrative medicine could do better than official medicine was unacceptable to them. It was a clash between the established medical system with its patented, synthetic drugs and a more natural approach. Anything natural that works better than synthetic drugs is perceived as a frontal attack on the entire economy of pharmaceutical companies. This rings especially true in France, where the government has its say in all things economic. The products, the man who conceived them, and all the know-how surrounding them must be destroyed.

At the time, my father was operating the only independent research laboratory in France, located in Saint Prim, in the Burgundy region. He had moved there in 1988, at age 65, having reached the mandatory age of retirement for academics in France.

On October 9, 1996, exactly nine months after Mitterrand's passing, the French S.W.A.T. team (in French the "GIGN") showed up in Saint Prim at 6:00 a.m. with machine guns, dogs, and a helicopter circling the laboratory. The scene seemed surreal for this sleepy little town. My father was handcuffed unceremoniously while walls were checked for secret hiding places. All products, samples for analysis, laboratory notebooks, letters, and research papers were seized. A moving truck was brought in to carry away computers, copy machines, and all raw materials, without even bothering to make an inventory of what was being taken away. The operation "ISA 2" was classified top secret, and those guys did not belong to the justice system at all, but to the military. Go ask a machine gun to show its warrant!

The GIGN made scores of arrests. There were about 700 doctors and several pharmacists working closely with my father at the time, and with more energy and determination than was ever used to chase down a dangerous gang of drug dealers, the GIGN searched the homes of all individuals who they suspected of using the products or being involved in their distribution. My brother's home was ransacked in front of his wife and children. The same would have probably happened to me, if I had not already been living in New York at the time. I learned that thousands of people in the following weeks took to the streets of Paris and other cities of France to show their support for my father and ask for free access to his botanical extracts. But the political power was stronger than the power of the street, and so the marches (and the marchers) were simply ignored.

It was at this point in telling my story when, finally, the computer and the projector arrived.

I had begun telling the audience this true-life drama merely to keep them from walking out, but during my talk something more had happened, something bigger.

I felt the audience was captivated by the action-packed scenario I relayed. Before beginning to present my slides, I had to complete my story.

I quickly told them the three things I promised my father on his deathbed:

1. To take the case, on his behalf, to the European Court of Human Rights.

2. To make sure the products would continue to be available.

3. To continue to do research with those extracts because the research validates their quality.

I explained that this, my last promise, is why I was now standing in front of this audience, scheduled to give a conference on cancer!

By then I had only twenty minutes left to talk about the research. I was extremely eager to present the valuable data, especially the stem cells study, so I quickly led them through the research conducted at KUMC by Drs. Qi Chen and Jeanne Drisko. These doctors have been interested in ovarian as well as pancreatic cancer and have explored the potential of Beljanski's botanical extracts as alternative therapeutic agents for these cancers.

As I mentioned earlier, both pancreatic and ovarian cancers are often frequently diagnosed late, develop drug resistance, and are similarly difficult to treat. Studies were first performed on cells, then on mice. The results[5,6,7,8] revealed the following:

- The extracts are nontoxic to ordinary human cells.

- The extracts have a selective effect against several lines of cancer cells.

- The extracts work in synergy with chemotherapies.

- Regarding the effect on ovarian cancer:

    o The conclusion was that "*In vivo, Pao pereira* (*Geissospermum vellosii*) alone suppressed tumor growth by 79 percent and decreased volume of ascites (the excess accumulation of fluid in the abdominal cavity) by 55 percent. When *Pao pereira* was combined with Carboplatin, tumor inhibition reached 97 percent and ascites was completely eradicated."

○ Combining *Rauwolfia vomitoria* with Carboplatin (a chemotherapy drug) remarkably enhanced the effect of Carboplatin and reduced tumor burden (the amount of cancer) by 87 percent to 90 percent and ascites volume by 89 percent to 97 percent.

▪ Regarding the effect on pancreatic cancer:

○ *Pao pereira* alone suppressed pancreatic tumor growth significantly, by up to 72 percent in mice.

○ As the tumors did not respond to Gemcitabine (another chemotherapy drug), the combination of Gemcitabine and *Rauwolfia vomitoria* significantly inhibited tumor progression. Notably, there were two mice that experienced complete tumor regression.

I could tell that my audience was impressed. They knew that if similar results were presented by a pharmaceutical company promoting a synthetic compound, such results would be published with great acclaim in *The Wall Street Journal*. But because there is no money in natural extracts, it is certainly a privilege to have this information available at all.

I moved on quickly to the cancer stem cells, my *pièce de résistance*. I was presenting data showing that those extracts, the *Pao pereira* and the *Rauwolfia vomitoria*, harmless to healthy cells, were both able to completely eradicate ovarian and pancreatic cancer stem cells! Sure, it was preliminary data, just done on cells, and had yet to be confirmed in an animal study, but I was so proud, almost intoxicated, with those results!

Silence set in.

"I have just time for one question," I finally said. There was another huge silence that felt like a century. Then one woman, seated in the front row, leaned forward and eagerly asked: "So how did you learn about the arrests? You said that you were in New York."

I was baffled. I had expected questions about the research that could possibly save their lives, not about my personal story. But I realized that my story was what captivated them. For years, my purpose for giving these presentations was to serve something bigger than myself, and advancing this beautiful research to fight cancer. And then, the one question that came up was not about cancer at all but about me ... *as if my story mattered.*

CHAPTER TWO
DESTRUCTION

"It is frequently the tragedy of the great artist, as it is of the
great scientist, that he frightens the ordinary man."

LOREN EISELY

S urprises come in many forms, so they say. Nonetheless, I was totally taken
off guard by the surprise in the form of a question on that beautiful
Sunday afternoon on Long Island.

"So how did you learn about the arrests?" the woman had asked. "You said
that you were in New York."

Yes. I was in New York and I was calling my father to see how he was doing....

The phone rang once, twice, three times. No answer. I thought it strange, but
decided to try back in an hour. It had become my practice to call my father
on a regular basis to check on him and see how his research was going. It was
my way of trying to connect with him since nothing else seemed to captivate
his interest.

This particular morning, October 9, 1996, was very different ... no one
was answering the phone.

It was unusual because there was always someone at the laboratory, and
I was always able to reach someone, if not my father himself. With the time

difference, it was the middle of the afternoon already in France and somebody should have answered.

After calling the laboratory several times and still not reaching anyone, I decided to call my mother at home.

The phone rang and a rather husky voice answered saying, "Hi."

I did not recognize it as my mother's voice, but who else could it be?

I responded hesitantly, "Mom? What happened?"

The voice replied briskly, "This is the police. Your mother is under arrest. You cannot speak to her."

I was stunned, but without taking the time to process this so-unlikely piece of information, I automatically went into "lawyer mode."

"I am a lawyer," I burst out, "and I would like to speak with my client."

There was an everlasting silence before I heard, "Okay, I'll give you two minutes."

I didn't know just how quickly two minutes could pass until that call. Within two minutes I was able to learn that my mother was physically fine and that she had no idea why she was arrested. Five men had been turning the apartment upside down since 6:00 a.m. without telling her what they were looking for, and she had no idea what was going on with my father. And she had not asked for a lawyer.

"I do not need a lawyer," she protested, "There is no need for the expense when I know I have done nothing wrong."

Without discussing the matter any further, I told my mom to hand the phone to the police officer. I asked him what the charges were, and he started to read over the phone a litany of charges—all about the promotion of unlicensed drugs and deception about their properties. I knew immediately that the "deception" charge could trigger jail time. The matter had to be taken seriously. I asked what the next step was going to be for "my clients." The officer said that he was not in charge of my father and could not provide any information about him, but my mother was going to be taken to jail and would be presented to a judge within forty-eight hours. I asked for his name and told him that "one of my colleagues" would contact him "quickly" to formalize my mother's legal representation.

We hung up.

I had butterflies in my stomach, but at the same time felt paradoxically calm. With Paris six hours ahead of New York, I knew that I did not have the luxury of panicking. Immediate action was the only way forward.

With a trembling hand, I reached for my agenda. I had been in New York for over a year working in a commercial law firm, and had no close contact in the criminal field. Yet here I was, seeking help for my own parents in something that was, undoubtedly, a criminal case.

I called my friend and colleague Marie-Odile Genefort, a family lawyer in Paris with great compassion and a strong work ethic. She immediately accepted my request to take care of my mother's immediate needs, and use all legal resources to inquire about my father's fate, which was, I was later to learn, an arrest as well.

I was extremely grateful for Genefort's support. I desperately needed help to work through this uncalled for, and largely unexpected, situation. As I later learned more about the circumstances of my father's arrest, I became aware of a very strange development...

Generally, according to French law, when policemen come to arrest you, they present you with their warrant and take you away. You are sent to jail and presented before the judge within forty-eight hours, as was the case with my mother. But instead of following this procedure with my father, the military men who came for him (not the police—a curious thing) did not present any warrant prior to ransacking the laboratory. They did not even have a specific list of persons to arrest. They simply proceeded to arrest all employees of the laboratory as they showed up for work.

My father was 73 at the time and never considered resisting the arrest. But instead of transferring him, without delay, to a judge for proper interrogation, they chose to interrogate him on the spot, without the presence of a lawyer. And while they interrogated him in one room, they sent for more men, who came into the laboratory covered from head to toe in white garments, looking like astronauts ready to walk on the moon. These men—I was told later by other employees who had also been arrested and witnessed the entire scene—began to spray the laboratory, claiming they were concerned about some possible radioactive activity, which made absolutely no sense whatsoever. Then again, instead of taking my father to the judge immediately, they said they would take the train to Paris the next day. They made him wait the day out in the laboratory, forcing him to spend the night exposed to the chemicals they had just sprayed.

To this day I don't know what was sprayed, what my father was exposed to, and I could never find anything in the legal file referring to the chemical spray or any basis for the so-called fear of radioactive components in the laboratory.

Eventually, my father was presented to the judge, and after a less-than-fifteen-minute hearing, he was sent home "under house arrest." He never even saw a jury. My father was required to surrender his passport, and was specifically forbidden to continue any kind of scientific research or to speak to journalists, even to merely respond to the negative stories issued by government-controlled press.

Shortly after his arrest, my father became very, very sick. Two months later, after being transported to the emergency room, he was diagnosed with acute myeloid leukemia, a disease that commonly spells rapid death for people over seventy.

My father had always been a strong and healthy man, while acute myeloid leukemia is believed to take decades to form. I couldn't help wondering... Could my father have been poisoned?

On top of my father's illness, the prosecutor in charge refused to properly instruct and prepare the case for trial. As a lawyer, I was absolutely shocked to see there was no due process given. Due process, according to French Law, in accordance to the French Constitution, guarantees that all legal proceedings will be fair and that an individual will be given notice of such proceedings and an opportunity to be heard within a reasonable time frame, before the government acts to take away their liberty or property (life is not an option, as the death penalty has long been abolished in France).

But this was not the case with my father versus the French government. The prosecutor was sitting on the case, denying all requests for hearings and expertise.

I was flabbergasted. I knew that my parents were looking to me to lead the defense team—even if it was remotely from New York—and each baseless refusal from the court felt like my own personal failure. I was crushed, shamed by the game that the French justice system was playing, and felt guilty for not winning their game.

At first, I couldn't even seriously consider the idea that my father had possibly been poisoned. It was just too much to process. Deep down, I felt there was something bizarre about the whole situation, but I couldn't comprehend the depth of it all. And I didn't want to believe it. But with the judge denying every hearing our lawyer requested, I knew that something was extremely and horribly wrong.

When I was finally able to access my parent's legal file, I was shocked by what I found.

Right there, in the legal file, there was a recommendation for the destruction of all evidence and testimonials of witnesses who had spoken highly of my parents or the products they created.

Justice is supposed to be about conservation of the evidence, not its destruction. But there it was. Clearly written. Black on white. With the signature of the officer in charge: "Recommendation of the destruction of all evidence and testimonials."

It was then I realized that the case wasn't really about bringing a man to justice, but about wiping out something that could make a significant difference for mankind. If the written order went so far as to include the destruction of all the related products and science, it's not far-fetched to imagine there was probably an unwritten order for the destruction of the man himself, hence the poisoning.

My father was dying at home and my mother nursing him day and night. The tragic irony was that none of his products were available to him because everything had been seized. The products he had been perfecting for years and that helped so many people couldn't help him in his own time of need.

In a desperate, heroic attempt to help my father, I proclaimed, "Do not die, Dad. I will make the products."

Obviously, I had no idea what I was getting into. I had no idea how to make the products, where they would come from, what herbs to use, how to sort them... I knew nothing. This is the point where I learned that the legal case had extended to all my father's suppliers as well, including the extraction and encapsulation companies. No one in France wanted to touch those products. They were all terrified of the repercussions, not even willing to return my calls.

I turned to my mother for guidance in trying to understand the products. She didn't have all the production details (it wasn't her specialty), but she could at least explain the original science that led my parents to start manufacturing in the first place. She could describe what was so unique and original about my father's research.

She explained that in 1965, the Nobel Prize in Physiology or Medicine had been awarded to three French scientists, all from the Pasteur Institute: François Jacob, Jacques Monod, and André Lwoff. They received the prize for their model of genetic regulation (the processes in the body that tell a gene when to "turn on" or express its specific characteristics). According to these highly-respected scientists, regulatory proteins control cellular processes by acting as on/off switches for gene expression.

That Nobel Prize established Monod as a famous scientist. In his highly publicized 1970 book *Chance and Necessity: An Essay on the Natural Philosophy of Modern Biology*[1], Monod concluded that all life and intelligence are only the result of natural processes that occur by "pure chance." He claimed that humankind is only the product of chance genetic mutations.

Monod asserted, "Pure chance, absolutely free but blind, at the very root of the stupendous edifice of evolution: this central concept of modern biology is no longer one among other possible or even conceivable hypotheses. It is today the SOLE conceivable hypothesis."

He later added "The universe was not pregnant with life nor the biosphere with man. Our number came up in the Monte Carlo game."

As with any game, there must be winners and losers. According to Monod's model, when it comes to life, chance mutations are the driving force for both good and bad. Chance mutations are the cause of evolution, but many mutations will hurt rather than help. If mutations are the only game in town, they may give us all that is great, but they are also responsible for the diseases that afflict us—like cancer.

Monod's assertion was important, and not purely scientific or even philosophical. Sold to the public and politics with proper media hype, this "mutational theory of cancer" was going to bring in big money in terms of research contracts and state subsidies. Soon, the "in vogue" concept of cancer was tied to the understanding of the genetic code and the central role of mutations, which meant that genetic therapies represented the "politically correct" bright future of medicine. (It always amazes me how political correctness is used again and again to stifle the emergence of any other valid scientific concept. Looking more closely, it appears that a dominant group often defines political correctness in order to serve its own political or economic agenda).

A mutation signifies change. In genetics, that means a change in the sequence of DNA in a cell. Think of DNA as the sentences in a very large book. The cell reads these sentences and uses the information to make proteins that control the behavior of the cell. Mutations change the letters in the sentences; thereby changing the information. The cell responds by making a defective protein. It is those altered proteins that cause cancer.

Through his research, however, Beljanski had the intuition that mutations were not the only kind of change in DNA that could lead to cancer. He saw how the famous double helix—the two strands of DNA wrapped around each other—is vulnerable to destabilization.

What is DNA destabilization?

The DNA's double helix is held together by fragile chemical bonds. These bonds stabilize the double helix, but they must be flexible so the cell can open the double helix to read genetic information and make copies of the DNA. The normal opening and closing of the DNA is tightly regulated in the cell.

Beljanski realized that molecules from our environment could influence the DNA structure and that some of these molecules (carcinogens) could destabilize the DNA by breaking the fragile bonds and separating the two strands of the double helix. In that case, the cell loses its control of DNA structure—the duplex is opened—and both gene expression and DNA duplication are no longer regulated.

Beljanski speculated that cancer cells divide continuously precisely *because* carcinogens have destabilized their DNA. In his laboratory at the Pasteur Institute, he compared the structure of cancer DNA with the structure of healthy DNA: the cancer DNA was more open! It was, in fact, destabilized.

He went on to demonstrate that the primary difference between normal and cancer DNA actually lies in the increased opening between the two strands of the double helix. In his view, mutations certainly can, and do, contribute to cancer, but they are secondary. Indeed, mutations are more likely to occur once the DNA has been destabilized, making the destabilization the primary factor.

Beljanski had provided environmental medicine with a scientific explanation at the cellular level on how the environment affects our DNA. Monod knew immediately this wouldn't go down in history as a simple battle of experts fighting to find the cause of cancer. Beljanski's approach had sound scientific backing, as well as philosophical consequences.

It was during that same time period that Beljanski did the "unthinkable": he dared question the "central dogma" of DNA supremacy and the notion that genetic information could only go from DNA to RNA.

The central dogma was defined by Francis Crick, who together with James Watson discovered the double-helical structure of DNA in 1953. It states that genetic information flows in one direction: from DNA to RNA. Monod had adopted it as the cornerstone of his doctrine and he was an absolutist: "It is neither observed nor indeed conceivable, that information is ever transferred in reverse" that is, from RNA to DNA, wrote Monod.[1] But my father's research continually proved the opposite. Beginning in 1969, Beljanski published several papers showing that RNA could very well carry information to DNA—the opposite of what Monod had asserted.

Monod was quite upset in 1971 when Dr. Howard M. Temin, an American scientist, discovered that a virus could have RNA as its genome (a complete set of genes). That discovery is important because it was thought, until then, that only DNA could contain a complete set of genes. In addition, Dr. Temin, discovered that this RNA genome specified an enzyme called reverse transcriptase which was capable of copying RNA into DNA. The discovery of that enzyme explained how a virus with an RNA genome (such as Hepatitis C or Herpes simplex) could integrate a DNA copy of its genome into the cellular DNA.

Monod hoped that this finding was an anomaly that would concern only the viral world, but it was soon to have far-reaching effects, because reverse transcriptase was the enzyme that would become associated with HIV, the human immunodeficiency virus that causes AIDS. (The discovery of reverse transcriptase is now considered one of the most important developments in the modern era of medicine. That fact, however, would not become evident for another ten years when the AIDS epidemic hit in 1981.)

Beljanski meanwhile continued his work, conscious that this was an extraordinarily promising field of research. In 1972, he discovered the existence of a reverse transcriptase enzyme in bacteria.[2] Bacteria are much bigger and far better organized organisms than viruses, and this was the first evidence of the importance of reverse transcriptase in the world of biology.

Monod, as Director of the Pasteur Institute, was extremely displeased and ordered Beljanski not to publish. Beljanski published anyway, and the rift between him and Monod became irreversible.

In 1974, Beljanski and his co-workers achieved the enzymatic synthesis of an RNA acting as primer in DNA replication. A "primer" is a short strand of either RNA or DNA that serves as a starting point for DNA synthesis and is required for DNA replication, making this an impressive discovery, especially since it was believed at the time that *only* DNA could act as a primer. Beljanski proved otherwise. Professor Pierre Lepine, Director of the Virology Department at the Pasteur Institute, announced Beljanski's result to the Academy of Sciences with a trembling voice, knowing full well the controversial impact the information would have. There was no looking back.

Temin was awarded a Nobel Prize, shared with David Baltimore, in 1975, and Monod made sure that Beljanski's work on reverse transcriptase would be forever buried (which it effectively was until 1989 when Temin recognized Beljanski's work in a retro citation published in *Nature*).[3]*

Nowadays, Monod's reductionist view that DNA "determines" just about everything in the entire organism has lost its appeal. It is even considered "dogma" (defined as a set of principles laid down by an authority that is considered true but may not necessarily be so). And dogma, in science, has, thankfully, become controversial. As biologist and philosopher James A. Shapiro put it, "The idea of a 'dogma' in science has always struck me as inherently self-contradictory. The scientific method is based upon continual challenges to accepted ideas and the recognition that new information inevitably leads to new conceptual formulations."[4]

Beljanski's challenge to the dogma of DNA and the destabilization model showing the susceptibility of DNA to the chemicals that surround us—which has since been independently confirmed[5]—are the two main reasons why my father is now often referred to as the Father of Environmental Medicine.

But that was not the end of the story.

After my father had figured out the link between environment and cancer, he wanted to test some molecules from the environment to see if they had carcinogenic potential. He developed a test that he called the Oncotest,[6] and started to analyze a number of molecules for their carcinogenic potential. The Oncotest revealed

---

* See Appendix 4: Retrocitation by Dr. Howard M. Temin

that it was environmental toxins causing the DNA to become destabilized. In other words, those carcinogenic toxins could cause the potentially deadly increase in the rate of cell division, even without the intervention of genetic mutation.

Beljanski was somewhat naïvely optimistic about the way the world operates. He thought industries that made food and personal care products would love his Oncotest: a test that would tell manufacturers, in a mere matter of hours, if there was a carcinogenic compound in their product so they could remove it from the market.

Beljanski patented the Oncotest only to find out that no industry was interested in testing, and potentially recalling, their products! Although it described a very inexpensive, easy way to find out if a product contained carcinogenic molecules, no one picked up the patent.

The Oncotest was simply too efficient—and potentially very expensive for companies that didn't want to change their products. The Ames test, considered the "best" test for carcinogens, remained unchallenged, even though it was much less accurate than the Oncotest.

Despite the resistance to his Oncotest, Beljanski continued his research. Next, as a true environmentalist, he reasoned that if nature could produce carcinogens, nature probably could produce anti-carcinogens. He decided to put the Oncotest to use testing if natural molecules had any selective anti-carcinogenic properties. In his search for specific compounds able to selectively block the duplication of cancer DNA, and leave alone the duplication process of healthy DNA, he discovered and perfected his *Pao pereira* and *Rauwolfia vomitoria* extracts.

The success of those extracts, confirming the theory that led to their discovery, was the supreme insult to the governance of the Pasteur Institute. With Monod's passing in 1976 (ironically, from cancer), and Beljanski now perceived as partly responsible for the crumbling of the central dogma of DNA, the senior scientists of the Pasteur Institute teamed up to portray Beljanski as a renegade scientist and sought to destroy his scientific credibility.

In 1978, Beljanski was forced to leave the Pasteur Institute. Passionate about his findings, my father continued his work at the Chatenay-Malabry School of Pharmacy, where he benefited from his knowledge of cellular regulation to test his extracts on animals and verify their safety and efficacy. By 1988, at the age of 65, he officially retired from academics. That's when he created his own laboratory in

Saint Prim and continued publishing until the fateful day that the army came to put a stop to his research.

Listening to my mother's explanation gave me a deeper appreciation of the brilliance and originality of my father's research. I also started to realize the importance of what my parents were doing. I could see that they were not more available to me when I was growing up because they were working on something tremendous: the acceptance of environmental medicine. Anger, frustration, resentment, and my highly prized self-pity, all the familiar feelings that I had nurtured for so long, began to fade away. I started to realize that it was not that I had been invisible to my parents. They had done their very best all along. Once I understood that, forgiveness came easy and instantly. It was as if a large, heavy weight had been lifted from my heart, and realization and relief flooded my being. I was not alone. I was part of a tribe, a family of which I could be proud.

If I had been committed to helping my father before, those scientific explanations my mother shared solidified my resolve. But even though the science was superb and did wonders for my spirit, it could not help me find the products or teach me how to make them. I knew that my father needed them fast if he was going to recover, but I had no idea where to turn.

In December 1996, two months after my father's arrest I was feeling somewhat desperate, and was nowhere close to finding any raw material, let alone someone to produce the botanicals, when I received a phone call from France.

"Hi, my name is Bernard Fourche," the mysterious caller explained in low tones, "I used to work with your father. I have been told that you are looking to make the products. Is this true?"

I replied cautiously, "... Yes ... Why? ... Do you have some products?"

Fourche spoke again and did I imagine, or did his voice drop even lower? "I cannot tell you anything over the phone, but I just wanted to know if you would be in New York next week and if I can meet with you."

"Of course. Of course ... Let me know when you are here."

A week later, Bernard Fourche came to New York. We met and he explained, "My company used to do the extraction process for your father. Then the army came and seized all the raw material and all the finished products. But they did not look into the machines, at what was actually being processed at the time of the raid. I have several hundred liters of *Pao pereira* extract, purified *Rauwolfia vomitoria* extract as well as golden leaf *Ginkgo biloba* extract available to you if you want them... Do you want them?"

I actually laughed out loud. I couldn't believe it.

I said, "Yes. Yes, of course, I want them but... I don't know how to treat them. I don't know how to dry them, I don't know how to encapsulate them, and I don't have money to pay you."

"Well, there is nothing I can do in France to help you with drying or encapsulating them. All I am offering is to ship you the liquid extracts. I'm going to ship you the entire inventory. I do believe that you will do something helpful with that and I trust you will pay me when you can. You are Mirko Beljanski's daughter. I trust you."

This man I had never met before, never seen, was stepping out of the shadows to help me!

I needed to call my mother at home in France, but I knew that the telephone was tapped. I didn't want to give the name of the gentleman over the phone and I couldn't say that I was going to receive hundreds of liters of extracts of each product. I only asked my mother to send me all the documentation she could find—notes and articles regarding the testing process, extraction process, all the toxicity studies—anything and everything she could find concerning the manufacturing of the products.

A few weeks later, I received a phone call telling me that the extracts were at Newark International Airport. A total of twenty huge barrels had escaped the vigilance of the French army and had been loaded on a train, a plane, and all the way through tough airline customs, all to be delivered to me! It was unbelievable.

What am I going to do now? I thought as I was tipping the Newark cargo freight employee to help carry the barrels to the back of a rental truck.

I had to find American companies able to dry and encapsulate the material.

In the meantime, not much was happening in France concerning my father's legal file. One full year after the arrest, no progress had been made with the criminal case. The prosecutor had finally agreed to appoint a panel of experts to analyze if the products seized were in conformance to their labels, but once the panel affirmed their conformity, he did not dismiss the "deception" charge. Instead, he did nothing to prepare for trial and provide my father with his fair day in court.

By 1997, my father was very sick and emotionally exhausted, and we both knew that asking him to stick around to help me was simply asking him to defy all odds.

"I will do my best," he said, "but it is very difficult to stay home all day, unable to work, to defend myself, to publish my last results... Life like that does not make sense anymore... I feel that I still have so much to say, that I could still contribute to..."

I was disheartened.

And then, as I closed my eyes, in a flash, the solution appeared to me.

In the legal tradition of modern democratic states, a basic requirement of the rule of law is that which is not expressly forbidden by law is permitted. The judge had expressly prevented my father to speak to journalists, but had said nothing about appearing in a movie. Therefore, nothing legally prevented Beljanski to speak in front of cameras and have his message recorded! And I just happened to have the right connections. Having paid my way through law school by lending my voice to many documentaries, recording radio commercials, and dubbing movies, I had friends in the industry. I had even dated a movie director for a while, and we had remained on good terms. Without hesitation, Philip accepted the challenge. "Finally, I'll get to meet your father!" he joked.

Obviously, there was no budget for a movie, but with a minimalistic camera crew and a black curtain for the only backdrop in my parents' own living room, he managed to give my father the opportunity of his last, long, uninterrupted interview.

Soon after, possibly emboldened by his stint before the camera, my father asked me if there was anything I could think of as a lawyer to speed up the resolution of the legal case, and I told him the only thing I could think of was to take the case before the European Court of Human Rights. "We have to do it" he said.

Once again, I committed to the task.

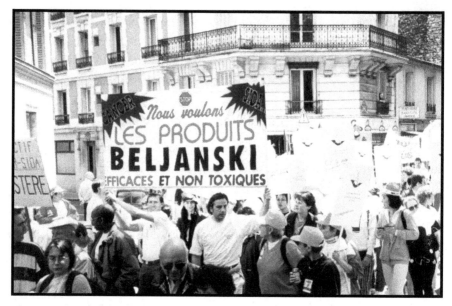

"We want the Beljanski products: efficient and not toxic" - Beljanski's supporters marching in the streets of Paris, 1997. (Photograph: Monique Beljanski - © The Beljanski Foundation, Inc.)

As I was actively battling the French government, I was also selecting American companies able to dry and encapsulate what I was now referring to as *"my extracts,"* and trying to send the capsules as quickly as I could to my father, hoping it was not too late. By this time, he was back and forth between the hospital and home.

In the meantime in Paris and other cities in France, loving supporters, outraged by the legal conundrum, organized petitions and marches, demanding my father's release and free access to his products. Thousands of people showed up to protest, but the press barely even reported it.

In 1998, while still stalling the criminal case and refusing to give my father his day in court to prove himself innocent, the French government decided to open up a tax case against him. The tax case was more legal nonsense—unless the intent was harassment and inducing a level of stress that would speed up the progression of my father's disease (when the defendant dies, the prosecutor no longer has to prove his case since the case is automatically closed). Killing the defendant is actually the best way for the government to close a case which would otherwise be impossible to win.

Indeed, between the criminal case and the tax case, my father felt completely harassed, and his health rapidly spiraled downward.

By the time we were trying to get in front of the European Court of Human Rights,* my father was becoming extremely ill and I had a feeling that the end was near.

With that in mind, I took a trip to Paris...

My legs felt like lead as I walked down the carpeted hallway and approached my father's bedroom. I wasn't quite sure what to expect as he had been bedridden for some days. I hesitated outside the door. I could hear him breathing. Slowly, laboriously, intensely... I knocked softly and slowly pushed in the heavy door. I stopped in the doorway, shocked. I couldn't believe what I saw. An old man lay on the bed. An old, bald, sick-looking man—just like the old men that would invade our apartment when I was a little girl. This could not possibly be my father. As though he felt my intense gaze, the old man opened his eyes and my heart melted. I recognized those eyes. They were just as bright and fiery as ever. And then he spoke, "Sylvie, you came."

The last day I went to see my father before flying back to New York, we both knew it would be the last time.

"I have to go back to New York," I told him. "I have my ticket for today... I wanted to tell you that I love you before I leave."

My father looked at me intensely for a moment and then said, "God bless you."

I couldn't hide my surprise.

Where did that come from? I had not been raised in a religious family. *We did not go to Church. We were basically a European agnostic family like most families in Europe...*

---

* It took us four years to get a decision, as the French government pulled every possible excuse, however poorly drafted, to delay the case. My father passed away in 1998—without a trial date ever set by the French judge—and we continued the case before the European Court of Human Rights on behalf of my mother. To this day, I am still shocked by the way the French government operated; in fact, I remain ashamed for the nation.

Eventually, in 2002, the long-awaited response came from the European Court of Human Rights. In a unanimous decision—Beljanski vs. France—the court recognized that France had no excuse for the numerous delays and for not giving my father his due day in court. We won. There was very little monetary compensation, but that's the way it is with the Court of Human Rights. Anyway it was not about the money. It was about the promise I had made to my father to find closure for the absence of the due process in France.

He continued, "God bless you. Don't change anything about the products and you will be fine."

And then he repeated, "God bless you."

I was shocked and I wasn't sure what to make of his blessing. Was I receiving the blessing because of my commitment to carry on the mission of manufacturing his products? Was my father finally seeing me and blessing me out of a love that had always been there, but he had been unable to express until the last moment—literally? On one hand, I felt I was given a purpose, a mission, but on the other hand, I could not help but wonder if my value as a human being was linked to my success with this mission.

Growing up, I had never been close to my father, but I can say that "thanks" to the legal issues we had grown closer in his last years. And now he was blessing me and giving me a mission. *Was my purpose on earth to fulfill this mission?* What I longed for so desperately as a little girl was wrapped up in those three little words.

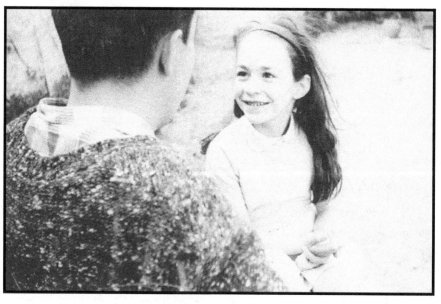

Young Sylvie Beljanski and her dad Mirko Beljanski (Photograph: Monique Beljanski - © The Beljanski Foundation, Inc.)

Mirko Beljanski passed away at home in Paris on October 28, 1998.

The city of Paris ordered for his burial three days after his passing—barely enough time to inform people, and definitively not long enough for organizing an autopsy ... another possible clue that there was something untimely with his passing.

Despite the last-minute announcement, a small crowd managed to come to the ceremony. A man came up to me to tell me that if it had not been for my father, he would never have been able to walk his daughter down the aisle.

"I would have never seen my grandchildren," said a breast cancer survivor woman.

"It is great that you carry on," said another.

I was proud, moved, and altogether overwhelmed.

At the cemetery, the air was cold and crisp. A helicopter was hovering, casting its noisy shadow above us. Coincidence? Maybe. The entire scene seemed surreal, and my recollection, tainted with emotion, is blurry. Except for the moment when a dark, tall, handsome man walked up to me.

"We have to talk," he whispered.

CHAPTER THREE
CIRIS AND THE BELJANSKI FOUNDATION

"Be the change you wish to see in the world."

Gandhi

I never would have thought something so tremendous would come from those few words whispered to me at the cemetery on that cold October morning. Or that Gérard Weidlich, a virtual stranger, would become such a key figure in my life. It just goes to show how strange and unpredictable life can be, and how, sometimes, we have to adjust ourselves to fit the bigger picture....

In the 1980s, a man approached my father, seeking a treatment that could help his child. His fifteen-year-old son had developed advanced leukemia, and, unfortunately, the boy's case was far too advanced for my father to help. This man nonetheless recognized that my father had something unique and valuable to offer humanity, and decided to help publicize his work however he could. Thus, CIRIS (Center for Information of Research and Scientific Innovation) a French nonprofit organization was created to:

1. Work towards the official recognition of the discoveries and innovative concepts developed by Mirko Beljanski.

2. Promote and coordinate the exchange of information, both nationally and internationally, related to the research and new treatments of diseases of cancerous, viral, or degenerative origin.

3. Spread awareness among patients, public organizations, and the media.

It was CIRIS that purchased a nineteenth-century run down winery in Saint Prim, Burgundy, that would become my father's private research lab. Thanks to the generous donations of the many individuals grateful to him for their restored health, a state-of-the-art laboratory was built within the old building. CIRIS had been a beautiful and flourishing nonprofit with several thousand members until 1996 when its headquarters were ransacked by the army and sealed by the marshals as a crime scene.

As a result of this judicial intervention, the CIRIS bank account was frozen. The magistrate responsible for freezing the account knew full well that a frozen bank account meant the inability of this otherwise rather healthy, and even wealthy, organization to pay its bills, leading to its subsequent and rapid dissolution. Sending CIRIS to bankruptcy court was just a clever way for the government to quickly shut down the laboratory and halt the flow of donations that were supporting Beljanski's research, while avoiding any and all public debate.

CIRIS was still in the midst of that situation when this man approached me at the cemetery, bending his towering figure to whisper in my ear. His initial words, "We have to talk," were followed by, "I am Gérard Weidlich, the President of CIRIS. You did promise to your father to continue, right?"

How he knew this, I did not know, but I quickly responded. "Yes. I haven't really figured out how I'm going to help, but I'm committed to do my best."

Gérard looked at me intensely, "Tomorrow at four at your parents' place."

"Excuse me?"

He repeated slowly, "Tomorrow at four at your parents' place."

By the way he spoke, I knew I had no choice in the matter. I had to be there.

So, at four o'clock the next afternoon, I found myself at my parents' apartment.

I hurried to open the door when I heard a knock, and if I was unnerved by the words spoken to me by Gérard the day before at the cemetery, it was nothing compared to what I felt when I opened the door. Gérard was standing before me, definitively intimidating, and flanked on one side by a pale, thin woman with white hair, and on the other, a tall, emaciated gentleman with lemon-colored skin.

A feeling of *déjà vu* came over me as I stood looking at this odd trio before me, and, for a second, I was back in my childhood.

Oh no, I thought, *these sick people are here for me now! How did that ever happen?*

And how was I ever going to get out of it?

I didn't know anything about science or about research, and I knew there was no way I could seriously help them. I didn't know why they even thought I could.

But I could not leave them standing at the door, nor could I close the door on them, so, as any polite hostess would, I invited them into the living room to sit down. There we were—Gérard, the pale woman, the lemon guy, and myself—sitting in my parents' living room, solemnly looking at one another. Gérard broke the silence.

"I have AIDS," he said.

I sure wasn't expecting to hear that, and I'm sure my surprise was written all over my face.

"It doesn't show," he explained, "Because I have been taking *Pao pereira*."

I was shocked.

Indeed, Gérard did not exhibit any of the side effects commonly associated with AIDS (Acquired Immuno Deficiency Syndrome) at that time: no weight loss, no visible red patches of the skin, no sunken eyes indicating chronic fatigue.

"I thought *Pao pereira* was for cancer," I replied.

"Not just for cancer. For viruses and different types of cancer."

He went on to tell his story.

Gérard was a lifeguard, and, one sunny day in the summer of 1985, he went to rescue a young man trying to drown himself in the ocean. He succeeded in bringing the young man back to shore, but he was not breathing well. Gérard attempted to administer mouth-to-mouth resuscitation, even though the man was vomiting blood.

A few months later, Gérard started to have fever, diarrhea, and other symptoms of illness. Since he was a strong and athletic former military officer who had never been sick, Gérard had some concerns, and went to see his doctor. The doctor ran tests and the result was HIV positive. In the pursuit of identifying when he had been contaminated, the doctor asked Gérard if he had been using drugs, and the answer was a resounding "no." In fact, Gérard was teaching classes against the use of drugs to teenagers as part of his line of work. It took him several weeks of trying to remember every detail of his recent activities before he would recognize when and how he had been infected.

At the time, there was absolutely no treatment for HIV (even AZT was not yet available*). The local authorities in charge of beach safety refused to recognize the HIV contamination as a result of a work-related incident, and therefore, Gérard was denied access to any kind of treatment through his insurance. He was on his own finding a solution for his situation, when his search led him to my father's publications.

"I am a father of four," Gérard told me, "I was not ready for a death sentence. I went to see your father and said I wanted to take *Pao pereira*. At first your father didn't want to hear any of it. He claimed that he could not do such a thing, that the extract had only been tested on mice, that there was a need for more studies."

Gérard told my father, "I have no time for more studies. The hospital wouldn't give me anything. I have nothing to lose. I beg you. I'll sign any waiver you want."

My father was known for being unable to turn down a man who had nowhere else to turn.

"I would not even know how much product would be needed for a big guy like you," my father objected, his resolve lessening with every word.

In the lab, the extract had shown to be very effective against many different viruses, including herpes, without side effects. But it had never been tested for AIDS. Would it be effective? Could it be possible that the very same extract already proven effective against so many kinds of cancer could also provide a solution for this terrible new disease?

"How much extract do you give your mice? I am 189 lbs. Let's do the math." said Gérard.

---

* Tri Therapy is now standard antiretroviral therapy (ART). According to the World Health Organization, ART consists of the combination of antiretroviral (ARV) drugs to maximally suppress the HIV virus and stop the progression of HIV disease. ART also prevents onward transmission of HIV. Huge reductions have been seen in rates of death and infections when use is made of a potent ARV regimen, particularly in early stages of the disease. "HIV/AIDS Treatment and Care." http://www.who.int/hiv/topics/treatment/en/. 11 November 2016

So, the two of them figured out the dosage, and Gérard started taking the *Pao pereira*. In a matter of months, all of his side effects (diarrhea, herpes, etc.) had disappeared. After a few years with the product, his viral load was completely undetectable. He credited *Pao pereira* for helping him maintain his flourishing good health and dashing good looks for the past thirteen years.[1]

"Don't you know that a clinical trial has been conducted on *Pao pereira* and HIV with very good results and has been published?"[2] he asked.

It suddenly came back to me. Actually it had been all that my parents seemed to have been able to talk about for at least two years! But I let him speak.

"I was doing so well that my family doctor could not believe his eyes. He wanted to know if I was an exception, or if this extract was going to be the next big medical miracle. He had good connections with a local hospital and started a clinical trial where HIV positive individuals took *Pao pereira* for one full year. It turned out that they all did quite well. Over the year their T4/T8 ratio (a test that shows how immunocompromised a person may be) improved instead of dwindling down. And it worked for all of them.

"But now, with the product being no longer available, I find my viral load is going up again." (Viral load is the measurement of the amount of a virus in an organism, typically in the bloodstream).

Was the same guy who had been begging my father some thirteen years earlier to save his life by giving him Pao pereira, begging me now to "do it again"? Seriously?

I ventured cautiously, "You are speaking of the same *Pao pereira* that was given to Mitterrand for his prostate cancer?"

"Yes, but it can do much, much more. It works on several kinds of viruses ... and plenty of different kinds of cancer."

"I am taking it for my breast cancer," interjected the pale woman. "Excuse me, I did not properly introduce myself. My name is Henriette Bouchet. Twelve years ago, I discovered a lump in my right breast. It first disappeared on its own, but in February of the following year showed up again."

I listened intently as she explained her situation.

In June of 1987, Madame Bouchet had a few tests done and learned she had a serious problem requiring surgery. After surgery, she was recommended to undergo the standard conventional treatment of radiation and chemotherapy. She became extremely sick and tired from the treatment, and knew that she would be unable to carry on with it much longer.*

"On July 9, 1988," Madame Bouchet stated, "I took charge of my life."

She decided to forgo any additional conventional treatments such as surgery, radiation, or chemotherapy, finding them full of damaging effects without any guarantee of extending her life. She then heard about Beljanski and a new concept of cancer causation, and opted to go this route instead.

As long as they had been available, she had been taking the *Pao pereira* and *Rauwolfia vomitoria* extracts, and had been doing remarkably well. However, since the products were no longer available, her markers were climbing. (Markers are substances found at higher than normal levels in the blood, urine, or body tissue of people with cancer. Markers are often used to track the progress of the cancer.)

Something about her speaking—whether it was the white hair or the deep wrinkles that ravened her cheeks—reminded me of my own grandmother. And then it hit me. Yes, when I was a teenager, Mamée, my beloved grandmother, had breast cancer, and yes, she turned down the surgery, as well as the chemotherapy. She claimed that she wanted to be a guinea pig for my father's products. My parents had done their best to convince her that there was a nice synergy of action between the extracts and chemotherapy or radiotherapy. They explained at length that she could have both, but to no avail. Grandma would not hear it. She chose to take the extracts only, and she survived her diagnosis for twenty-two more years, outliving my grandfather who never had cancer.

With my parents both busy making scientific history, my grandmother had been central to my upbringing. To this day, I miss her.

But there was no time for nostalgia. The lemon-colored man was speaking, cutting short my trip down memory lane.

"I have no right to ask for anything," he began, "But I am a father of five, and if you can help me with *Pao pereira*, I will be forever grateful."

His name was Jean-Paul Le Perlier, and he was a journalist. His first contact with Beljanski's research came in 1993 when he was assigned to write an investigative

---

*   For Henriette Bouchet's full testimonial go to www.beljanski.org and see also *Cancer's Cause, Cancer's Cure: The Truth about Cancer, Its Causes, Cures, and Prevention* by Morton Walker published by Hugo House Publishers, Ltd.

story against my father. (As President Mitterrand started to get better, journalists knew there was a story to be told).

My father had been described to him as a charlatan pretending to cure cancer and AIDS with some sort of mysterious concoction made from plants. Since there was no legal case or sound evidence against Beljanski, Le Perlier's job was to create a case by finding several victims of the supposedly medical fraud and interviewing them in an attempt to expose this great societal injustice. Despite months of diligent investigating, Le Perlier was not able to find anyone with complaints about my father and his work. Everyone he spoke to seemed quite pleased with the changes in their lives because of my father's "magic powder."

Finally, Le Perlier met a woman who claimed that she was very angry with Beljanski. That was music to his ears. At last, he was going to be able to write his long-overdue news article! However, upon further investigation, he discovered that the woman's disposition was due to the fact that her husband, who had been using the products faithfully, had recovered so well from his cancer, he had left her and took off with the neighbor. The scorned wife would have rather seen her husband die. She was as upset with Beljanski as she was with the other woman!

I asked Le Perlier, "So you were hired to demolish someone's character *before* actually researching his character?"

He shrugged and replied matter-of-factly "Yes. It happens all the time. The newspaper tells us what the narrative is, and then journalists have to come up with content that will fit that narrative. But in this case, the more patients and doctors I interviewed, the more convinced I became that I could not write the story as assigned."

He went back to his publisher and explained that, based on his investigation, the only story he could write about Beljanski was a positive one. He was told that the magazine had been commissioned by an anonymous source to run a negative article and that they would rather kill the story than run a positive one.

"Come up with something" urged the publisher.

Le Perlier, however, declined to lie about his findings. Shortly after, he was fired from his job, which was devastating for a father of five.

"And now I have advanced colon cancer myself," he continued. "I went to the most reputable specialists in Paris only to be told that the cancer has spread everywhere in the abdomen, that I have about three months to live, and they will be three months of hell. My wife has left me and I have five children at home. Do you think you can help me?"

I felt cursed: those sick people who used to go to my parents asking for help were now coming to me! But then again, how could I say no?

For the first time, I was putting myself in my parents' shoes. And then I remembered my father saying, "Whenever you can help, you have the duty of doing so."

I looked at those three miserable souls before me and felt the full weight of their burdens upon my shoulders.

"How did I ever get myself involved in this mess?" I thought.

Aloud I managed to articulate a more damage-controlled response. "If I help you and all three of you get better, will you help me to carry on? There is no way I can do this alone."

They swore they would help me in any way they could.

Gérard, a military officer at heart, immediately started to devise a plan of action. He explained that CIRIS had about four thousand members still willing to give money in support of the research, but now that my father was gone and there was no research project, no new money could be raised. Even finding the funds to pay for a lawyer who would fight CIRIS's freeze order in court was an issue.

"If there was a new research program announced in New York," he continued, "I could tell the members that the story is not over, do some fundraising, open a new bank account, hire a lawyer, get the bank account unfrozen, avoid bankruptcy court, keep CIRIS alive, and send you money to fund the research. All you have to do is to come up with the extracts, a research program, and a way to send us our treatments."

"All I had to do" sounded like a lot, but thanks to Bernard Fourche, I already had several kegs of extracts available. The whole thing was kind of a long shot, but what else could I do?

"Okay. We have a plan," I conceded.

We shook hands.

Gérard had now promoted himself to the rank of general, running an army of three.

"Henriette," he ordered, "You will find a way to get a hold of the list of all the people who have attended CIRIS's conferences over the past three years. They need to be informed immediately that we are back in business and the research goes on!"

Without waiting for an answer, he turned to the-ever-yellower-looking Le Perlier. "Jean-Paul, find Dr. Marcowith's widow. Convince her that we need all of his notes to continue, and bring back the manuscript—"

"Who was Dr. Marcowith?" I interrupted.

Gérard turned to me, "Dr. Marcowith was a very good doctor, and a friend of your father. His practice was just a few miles away from the laboratory in Saint Prim. He was one of our best lecturers. At the time of his sudden passing in 1996, Dr. Marcowith was writing a book and working on developing new avenues of research with your father."

And then, looking at me intensely, he added, "And you are going to continue all of this from New York."

He extended his hand. Once again, we shook hands.

Late that same evening, I asked my mother how the same product could be effective against viruses as well as so many different kinds of cancers.

"Your father worked a lot on enzymes," she began. "Before his discovery that reverse transcriptase was present in bacteria, it was only known to be in viruses. Beljanski's discovery of reverse transcriptase in bacteria was huge because bacteria are everywhere. The phenomenon that scientists had once thought to be contained to the viral world, was in fact, everywhere. Your father could have stopped his investigation there. But then AIDS appeared. In the beginning, nobody knew anything about it, and it was kind of a new plague. From 1981 through 1987, new HIV/AIDS cases and fatalities doubled roughly every year. The year 1987 saw forty-thousand deaths and nearly fifty-thousand new cases. Scientists were not sure about the way this deadly virus was transmitted, but that did not prevent them from giving all sorts of opinions and advice.

"In the meantime, both the Pasteur Institute in France and Abott Laboratories in the United States were racing each other to find a test to check if transfused blood was clear of the virus. Abott came first, and revealed that the virus could be destroyed by heating up the blood before transfusion. In France, the Pasteur Institute used all its political might to delay the approval of the American test, hoping to come up with their own in the interim. Knowingly, the heating process was not implemented, resulting in additional thousands of people contaminated with AIDS because of bad blood transfusions. It was a huge scandal. At the time, there was no treatment available and an AIDS diagnosis was equivalent to a death sentence.

"Always looking to help people, your father, once in possession of his unique plant extracts selected through the Oncotest, thought of studying their potential activity in inhibiting the virus's reverse transcriptase. He then discovered that his *Pao pereira* extract was very effective inhibiting the reverse transcriptase of several families of viruses whether RNA viruses (like the Herpes virus, Hepatitis C virus, and AIDS virus) or DNA viruses (Hepatitis B, for example)."

"And the Pasteur Institute did not welcome that discovery?" I asked.

"Quite the opposite" was her quick reply.

Many authors concur that AZT was, from the beginning, a very controversial drug. In 1964, a chemist, Jerome Horwitz, synthesized a sophisticated experimental cell poison for the treatment of cancerous tumor cells. It was called Suramin, or Compound S. Its formal title is 3'-azido-3'-deoxythymidine zidovudine, for short—but everyone knows it by its nickname, AZT. AZT disrupts DNA synthesis—a necessary function of every cell in the human body. It irrevocably scrambles the DNA code a cell needs to replicate. But that did not prevent the pharmaceutical company Burroughs Wellcome from quickly launching AZT on the market in 1987.

Anthony Brinks, an advocate of the High Court of South Africa and former prosecutor, described AZT as "A Medicine from Hell":

"That's the end of the cell line. Cell division and replication, wrecked by the presence of the plastic imposter, come to a halt. Chemotherapeutic drugs such as AZT are described as DNA-chain-terminators accordingly. Their effect is wholesale cell death of every type, particularly the rapidly dividing cells of the immune system and those lining our guts. Horwitz found that the sick immune cells went but with so many others that his poison was plainly useless as a medicine. It was akin to napalm-bombing a school to kill some roof-rats. AZT was abandoned. It wasn't even patented. For two decades it collected dust, forgotten—until the advent of the AIDS era."[3]

There was nothing on the market to address this new disease called AIDS, and political pressure from activists and lobbyists was mounting. Larry Kramer, an American playwright, author, and public health advocate, was especially vocal, giving impassioned speeches, deliberately defining AIDS as a holocaust (mainly due to the apathy he saw in the response with which the United States' government was expending the necessary resources to find a cure, which they were doing largely because AIDS mostly infected gay men and minorities).

Through speeches, editorials, and personal, sometimes publicized, letters to figures such as politician Gary Bauer, former New York Mayor Ed Koch, several *New York Times* reporters, and Anthony Fauci, the head of the National Institute of Allergy and Infectious Diseases, Kramer personally advocated for a more significant response to AIDS.

In 1987, Kramer was the catalyst in the founding of the AIDS Coalition To Unleash Power (ACT UP), a direct action protest organization that chose government agencies and corporations as targets to publicize lack of treatment and funding for people with AIDS. ACT UP was formed at what is now known as the Lesbian, Gay, Bisexual and Transgender Community Services Center in New York City, and quickly sprouted numerous "chapters" around the world.

The FDA, in the face of growing pressure, was desperate to approve "something." Celia Farber, an American journalist well known for having extensively written about HIV/AIDS recalls[4]:

"On a cold January day in 1987, inside one of the brightly-lit meeting rooms of the monstrous FDA building, a panel of 11 top AIDS doctors pondered a very difficult decision. They had been asked by the FDA to consider giving lightning-quick approval to a highly toxic drug about which there was very little information... But there were tremendous concerns about the new drug. It had actually been developed a quarter of a century earlier as a cancer chemotherapy, but was shelved and forgotten because it was so toxic, very expensive to produce, and totally ineffective against cancer. Powerful, but unspecific, the drug was not selective in its cell destruction."

AZT was approved in record time with only one trial on humans instead of the standard three, and that trial was stopped after nineteen weeks. From the onset, there was evidence of widespread collusion: none of the other drugs in development to fight AIDS were granted this same shortcut to approval. Instead, Burroughs Wellcome (since merged into GlaxoSmithKline) announced that it had been granted a monopoly on the drug's patent, and its cost would be upwards of $10,000 for a single patient annually, making it the costliest drug ever at the time, as reported by the *New York Times*.[5]

My mother continued:

"With our *Pao pereira* extract, we succeeded in having a clinical trial done at the hospital, and we expected that the results showing that it was very effective and very well-tolerated would be exciting news. It wasn't. While the clinical study investigators concluded that the product could be considered as a promising new drug for the effective treatment of HIV-1 infection,[2] no pharmaceutical company nor governmental agency was interested in developing a safe and natural answer to the problem.

"Since there is very little "big money" to be made with botanical solutions to cancer and other diseases, they are ignored in favor of money-making drugs, even if the botanical is shown to be more effective and far less toxic. Such was the case with AZT versus *Pao pereira*.

"With its toxicity coupled with an astronomical price, AZT was a very bad choice overall. Its damage to the organism was irreparable. But precisely *because* it was a very bad drug, its marketing had to be very effective. They enrolled activist groups like ACT UP to fight as 'quackery' anything that might have worked better than AZT. In France, Philippe Mangeot, who was running the national chapter of ACT UP, was none other than the son of Jean-Pierre Mangeot, President of Glaxo Wellcome France! There was no way they would have allowed a piece of their 'market share' to pass them by.

"ACT UP and the National Board of Pharmacy colluded their efforts to discredit your father. At every conference where he was speaking, ACT UP would send a group of all-black-dressed activists to disrupt the scientific discussion. They spread lies about Beljanski in the press, claiming that he was discouraging people to take their meds or was asking considerable amounts of money for his extracts. They claimed that there was no scientific evidence of the extract's effectiveness, while dismissing as "nonsense" all the evidence that did indeed exist. Anonymous sources made accusations of quackery, and claimed that the plant extracts were "mysterious" even though everything about them had been published. The witch hunt was not only directed against Beljanski. It was also directed against the few journalists who did not endorse the majority's views, and dared to be critical of AZT's obvious toxicity.

"Eventually, as the toxicity of AZT was becoming more and more apparent, it prompted additional studies. A 1993 French-British study of about 1,750 patients (termed the "Concorde" study after the cooperative development of the Concorde aircraft by Britain and France) showed that after an average of three years of treatment, the patients treated with AZT did not experience a longer AIDS-free period than untreated patients, but typically went on to develop one or several of the complications associated with AZT, such as anemia, bone marrow toxicity, and even lymph cancer (one of the most severe side effects of AZT is cell-depletion of bone marrow). That same year a National Cancer Institute study showed that people who took AZT for two to three years had a 49 percent incidence of lymphoma, compared with approximately 2 percent in AIDS patients not on AZT.[6]

"Finally AZT was about to become completely discredited, and the world was at last ready to look for an alternative, when Beljanski's laboratory was ransacked and everything came to a halt. I guess that no matter how toxic it may be, one can't take on the most expensive drug ever—there's just too much money involved!"

"So, is it fair to say that you and Dad were not only pioneers for cancer treatment, but also for AIDS treatment, and that the government would not hear any of it?" I asked.

"Yes, kind of," my mother answered softly.

"And what about the other extract, the *Rauwolfia vomitoria*? Does it also work against the AIDS virus?" I wanted to know.

"No," she replied. "The *Rauwolfia* did not exhibit any antiviral properties."

But then my mother dropped another bombshell on me, "The *Rauwolfia* extract that your father perfected does not have any effect on blood pressure because, in order to avoid toxicity, he made it reserpine free. It has a good anticancer activity, and it is very effective to help regulate hormones and boost fertility."

"Boost fertility?"

"Yes," she continued, "Actually there is a funny anecdote about it. We once helped a farmer suffering from advanced pancreatic cancer. He fully recovered and was looked upon as 'a miracle' by other surrounding farmers.

"The growing infertility of their pigs was creating serious hardship to the farmers living in that area. One day, we received a visit from a group of his neighboring farmers. They were inquiring if your father would perform another 'miracle', this time on their pigs, to get them to have more piglets. Mirko gave them some *Rauwolfia*, to feed both to the males and the females. We did not hear back from the farmers for several months until, one day, they came back with another complaint: "It worked too well... too many piglets and not enough nipples! Do you have something to develop more nipples?"

"Really?" I marveled. "Has it ever been used by people, for getting pregnant?"

"Oh, yes!" my mother exclaimed. "Pigs and humans are not different in that regard. With *Rauwolfia*, Dr. Marcowith helped a lot of couples who had problems to conceive. It was most special to your father to receive pictures of beautiful babies. Because of lack of time and resources, we did not publish on that topic, but it is hugely important. Everywhere there is a growing infertility issue linked to pollution."

Indeed, demographers such as Michael Teitelbaum at Harvard Law School, and Jay Winter, a history professor at Yale University, note that already more than half the world's population lives in aging countries where the fertility rate is less than 2.1 children per woman—the rate required to replace both parents once infant mortality is taken into account.[7]

And humans are not alone! Dr. Louis Guillette, an endocrinologist from the University of Florida, has spent the last decade studying the influence of environmental contaminants on fetal development and reproductive systems of wildlife and humans. He has studied the differences between alligators living in contaminated Florida lakes and those in cleaner ones. Alligators in Orange

County's very polluted Lake Apopka had on average 24 percent smaller penises than alligators in Lake Woodruff, which was chosen for study due to its relatively pristine nature as there is no agriculture or industry nearby and only a few residences directly adjacent to the lake.[8]

Historically, the 30,000-acre Apopka lake has been a dumping ground for DDT and other toxic materials, and its water quality worsened by agricultural discharges (runoff) and ineffective drainage. Dr. Guillette found 70 percent lower plasma concentrations of testosterone in Lake Apopka alligators when compared to animals of similar size on Lake Woodruff. Abnormal hormone levels like those are associated with decreased sperm counts and reduced fertility.

Pesticides, fungicides, heavy metals, defoliants, and other chemical weapons, in addition to oils and cleaning agents, are now regarded as the main environmental pollutants capable of disrupting spermatogenesis.[9]

When the time came for these juvenile alligators to reproduce, their significant reduction in penis size made it difficult to mate and "certainly didn't impress the lady alligators" the *Miami Times* reported, jokingly, at the time.[10]

But the issue was no joke. After the effect of contaminants on fertility became known, President Clinton and Congress moved to create legislation and called hearings where Guillette and others warned that reproductive malfunctions similar to the alligators' might well be in store for other creatures—including humans—owing to the polluted state of our planet.

"You are not half the man your grandfather was," Guillette told one legislative panel.

Indeed, a long-term Danish study has revealed that sperm counts in men around the world have decreased 50 percent over the past five decades.

"I testified before Congress and said that every man in the room was half the man his grandfather was, and everybody quotes that line," said Guillette. "But the question is, 'Will our grandsons be half the men we are? Will we face widespread infertility?"[10]

I knew I was entering uncharted territories, with an infinite realm of possibilities. I felt almost dizzy.

"Are you now claiming that you can save humanity from extinction?" I asked my mother.

"No, unfortunately, I would not go there," she replied. "But we have helped many desperate couples have children."

I leaned forward and looked at my mother intensively, wondering if I was exhausting her.

"One last question," I said, "How come the same extracts work on different kinds of cancer, like on Mitterrand's prostate and Mrs. Bouchet's breast? This is something completely unheard of."

"Indeed," she responded without hesitation. "Your father turned the whole understanding of cancer upside down. All the laboratories around the world work on the general and accepted assumption that cancer is caused by mutations. But mutations happen when there are changes in the genetic code. Instead your father observed that all cancer cells exhibit changes in their secondary DNA structure: the hydrogen bonds that hold the DNA strands together in a double helix are broken. This means that the strands of DNA are opened up, leading to a destabilization that allows the enzymes that copy DNA to work overtime. The DNA keeps duplicating, enabling cells to keep dividing without stopping. This is what happens to DNA in the presence of a carcinogen:

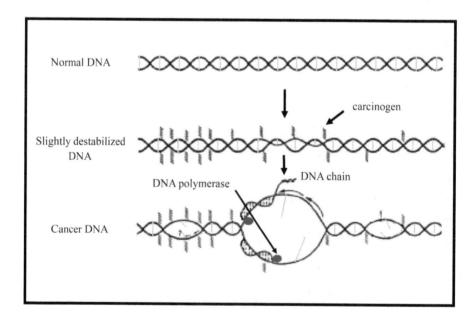

"At first, this destabilization is minimal, but if a cell is in continual contact with a carcinogen, the destabilization increases dramatically. Then the cells replicate much faster and in an unregulated manner. This is the high mark of cancer cells."

"The Oncotest revealed that many of today's chemicals act as carcinogens and induce different kinds of cancers. What your father also found is that some natural extracts are able to recognize destabilized DNA, and selectively block its ability to replicate. Those extracts are actually doing the exact opposite of carcinogens. Since they work on the level of the DNA, they are not organ- or gender-specific."

I knew that my mother was a research engineer, still I was really impressed with her knowledge, and grateful for her willingness to explain.

"At first, I was not specifically interested in biology, but working with your father has been fascinating," she went on to say. "And the more you learn and understand the science, the more fascinating it gets."

Two days later, I was back in New York, my head still spinning with all that I had learned.

I shared my Paris encounter with Ken, my husband at the time, who was a lawyer in New York with his own practice. I tentatively tried to explain that I was thinking of starting a research project in order to support a French nonprofit organization whose bank account had been frozen, and in doing so, we would save humankind.

The conversation did not go well.

"Are you completely out of your mind?" he practically yelled at me.

Well, I was beginning to wonder the same thing, but, of course, I couldn't let him know that. I braced myself and tried to ignore the comment.

"Could you please create a U.S. nonprofit organization for me?" I calmly asked.

While this request seemingly came out of nowhere, it actually came to me while I was flying home. I had a deep intuition that a U.S. nonprofit was the best way to carry on the research program, and, ultimately, my father's legacy.

"Sure, I could," he replied. "But this is going to be a lot of work, and you are not going to be able to do anything with it."

"Thank you," I was determined to ignore all negativity.

Three months later, the application for the U.S. nonprofit was still a non-starter, and after another three months, there was still no progress. By then, I had received from Gérard Weidlich and Henriette Bouchet the names and contact information for all the doctors who had been working closely with my father and attended lectures at Saint Prim.

I realized that if I was going to carry on my father's legacy and research program, it was important to establish a close network with all the doctors already familiar with his work. I had to meet them.

I decided I would rent a meeting room in a New York hotel and invite all of them to attend a "symposium" on Beljanski's research. To get speakers, I called the first five names on Gérard's list to introduce myself, and asked them if they would come to New York to lecture about my father's work. The response was unbelievably enthusiastic. They all told me they had long been waiting for such an opportunity.

One of the French doctors on the list wanted to know if the symposium would also be open to American medical doctors and medical journalists. I told her that I wanted to be as inclusive as possible, but that I did not know any people in these fields. She then revealed that, some twenty years earlier, she had a steamy summer fling with an American student attending the famous French Institute of Political Sciences (Sciences Po). The student was now a medical journalist, and the symposium seemed the perfect opportunity to reconnect discreetly. She gave me a Seattle phone number and instructed me to call "Pat."

Lucky for me, Pat seemed thrilled to hear a French accent on the phone.

"OUH, Anne-Marie, comment ça vaaa?"

I explained that I was not Anne-Marie, but confirmed Anne-Marie would love to see him in New York and asked if he would plan to attend the symposium. I had to promise that "to the best of my knowledge" Anne-Marie looked the same as she did twenty years ago, and that "I would do my best" to ensure that his torrid recollection would go untarnished. (Legal disclaimers are so handy!)

It did not take him long to clear his schedule.

"By the way," I added, "Do you know of any doctors who would be interested in attending?"

He gave me a short list of holistic doctors in the New York area that I could call on his behalf. One of them was Dr. Michael Schachter from Suffern, New York, an excellent doctor with lots of experience and known for his on-the-mark diagnoses. He is also a wonderful, generous, compassionate human being with a curious, open-minded spirit, always on the lookout for something that might help his patients. Little did I know at that time just how decisive that recommendation would become.

Finally, I announced to Ken that I had a symposium scheduled in New York with about a hundred doctors planning to attend, several speakers lined up, and that I was counting on him to officially announce the launch of the Foundation. He sighed.

"Okay. What do you want to call it?"

Without hesitation, I replied, "The Beljanski Foundation."

CHAPTER FOUR
THE SYMPOSIUM

"Just when the caterpillar thought the world was over,
it became a butterfly."

ANONYMOUS

S ometimes you have to put blinders on and push ahead with all your
might in order to get ahead in life. There will always be something,
or someone, standing in the way of where you need to go. The key is to
persevere and stay focused on the task at hand. Keep your eyes on the
goal. Although, sometimes you have to close your eyes and your ears, and just
trust your heart....

The response to the New York City symposium was incredible. It went far
beyond the initial list of French doctors provided by Gérard Weidlich. More
doctors, scientists, and even people with illnesses (having heard about the
symposium through the grapevine) were calling me from all over the world
asking if they could attend.

Of course, I said "yes" to everyone.

About ten days before the event, I received a note from Professor Shmuel
Shoshan, an Israeli scientist associated with Hadassah-Hebrew University
Hospital of Jerusalem. Interestingly, this ultra-modern complex, which includes schools of medicine, dentistry, nursing, and pharmacology springs
from an organization that was established in 1912 in New York City. Pro-

fessor Shoshan told me that he had learned about my father's work through Sten Friberg, a senior consultant in Oncology at Karolinska University Hospital in Stockholm and son of Stone Axel Friberg, former president of the Karolinska Institute and, from 1953, a member of the Nobel Foundation.

Indeed, I was aware that my father's work had been read with great interest at Stockholm's Nobel Foundation. In 1980, he even received a letter from Sten Friberg telling him, "Your ideas and results are simply fascinating," and asking him to send to Stockholm "copies of all papers and manuscripts dealing with those studies."* The Pasteur Institute, however, had made sure to cut off the Nobel Foundation's interest in any research related to Mirko Beljanski.

"Your father was a genius," continued Professor Shoshan. "The idea of cancer resulting from a progressive and cumulative destabilization of the DNA is revolutionary, and his work on oligoribonucleotides was absolutely unique. I have since 'devoured' all his publications I could gain access to. His work was truly brilliant. I am so sorry to hear that he passed away. I can just imagine the conversation that I could have had with him. Would you allow me to come to your symposium and salute his memory by presenting a retrospective of his work through his publications?"

My father left behind a body of 133 peer-reviewed papers.** I knew right away that Shoshan's presentation might possibly be the highlight of the symposium.

Since the schedule for the symposium was already looking pretty full, I decided to make it a two-day symposium. I made a note to check on this "oligoribonucleotides" thing later, and called the hotel to extend the reservation for an extra day.

Two days before the event, Gérard and his wife, the lovely Pierrette, arrived in New York. He had mysteriously told me over the phone that he had two surprises for me.

Not looking exhausted in the least by his seven-hour flight and six-hour jet lag, Gérard could not wait to share that a judge had finally ruled that there were no grounds to force CIRIS to file for bankruptcy when it had money in the bank. The judge had urged the prosecutor to provide legal basis for the freeze of the bank account or see the freeze order revoked.

---

*   See Appendix 5: Letter from Dr. Sten Friberg

**   See Appendix 1: Scientific Publications of Mirko Beljanski

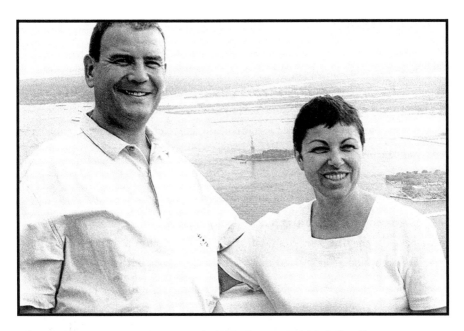

Gérard and Pierrette Weidlich in New York in 1999 (Photograph: Sylvie Beljanski)

And not only had the bank account been restored, but a number of documents seized from the laboratory had been returned.

"And now that I know that they acted without the proper warrants, I am going to fight to get back everything," Gérard exulted. "This is just the beginning!"

Proudly, he exhibited two folders: one that looked like a manuscript bearing my father's hand writing, and the other one a notebook labeled "Dr. Christian Marcowith." He also had a letter signed by Marie-Laure Marcowith (Dr. Marcowith's widow) bequeathing to The Beljanski Foundation all rights to the notebook.

What on earth am I going to do with them? I wondered. Although I had not the slightest idea what to do with these two items, I thanked Gérard profusely.

Now I was in charge of important hand-written documents that I could not even understand!

I decided to tuck them away in a safe place to try to decipher them later.

My mother arrived in New York as scheduled. I had not seen her in months, and the reunion, after all we had gone through as a family, was quite emotional. Her gentle eyes, usually clear and sharp, were clouded with layers of undisguised emotion. Her face, framed by soft, nearly-white curls, looked tired and worn, and her gait was noticeably slower. It was obvious that she had been badly shaken by the events in France, and her heart had been broken beyond repair. But, with the sense of dignity and privacy that defines her so well, she would not dwell on her feelings. Instead, she handed me some envelopes—unopened letters addressed to my father and received since his passing.

"Here are some things that may be of interest to you now," she said, reaching into her leather satchel for a few more items.

"We need to talk," I answered, knowing how this little sentence seems to always have the magic power of grabbing someone's attention. I was right. She immediately stopped what she was doing and looked at me with questioning eyes.

"I am not going to do this alone," I began boldly. "I am launching a foundation. You have to be the President of The Beljanski Foundation. You worked in the lab with dad for almost forty years. You have the scientific knowledge and the credibility. I'll sponsor you for a green card, but you have to come to New York. I can't do it without you."

Those cloudy, gentle eyes stared at me for a moment, and I felt ever so small. Not a word. Just a look, one that spoke volumes.

The older you are, the harder it is to start over in a new country with a new language, and my mother was almost sixty at the time. I could tell that she wasn't thrilled with the idea of leaving her settled life in Paris behind and moving to New York for good. Consternation was all over her face.

Was I being selfish in my selfless reach for the greater good? Was I too demanding?

At the same time, everybody seemed all right with requiring a piece of me without asking my opinion, I reasoned within myself. *Besides, her knowledge and expertise were essential to the success of whatever "it" was going to be.*

She took a deep breath and, after a long pause, whispered, "If that's what you want..."

Guilt immediately assaulted me.

"This is for the greater good," I replied.

I was trying to convince us both.

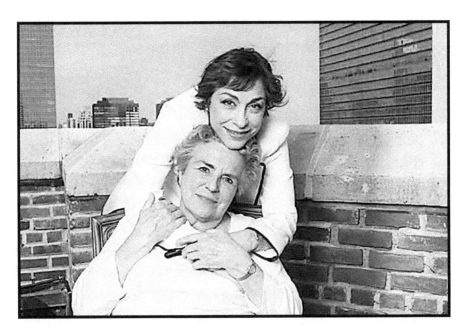

Monique and Sylvie Beljanski in New York (Photograph: John C. Cooper - © John C. Cooper)

September 25, 1999: the morning of the symposium arrived too soon, and I was a nervous wreck. But there was no turning back time. The day had come, and it was filled with buzz from the beginning. The French doctors arrived by the score. Some knew each other and some did not. Some knew me and some did not, but even those I had never met before endeavored to hug me, kiss me, or squeeze my arm, as a display of their genuine affection for the memory of my father.

Love was overflowing. It was love that felt, to me, like a down payment—one that you can start enjoying today but will still have to earn tomorrow. For that day, however, there was no time to nurture anxiety for the installments.

I spotted a gentleman looking surprised and somewhat lost in the middle of the French-speaking crowd, and walked over to him. Dr. Schachter has the face of goodness itself. I thanked him for coming and assured him there would be a translation service offered all day long. Then, as if on cue, Professor Shmuel Shoshan appeared, looking exactly as I had imagined him: an old, frail figure sporting a long grey beard with piercing blue eyes peering through round, gold-framed glasses. I introduced the two men — at least they could speak English to each other!

Pat, the medical journalist from Seattle, had taken a red-eye, and showed up soon after (I had the difficult duty of informing him that Anne-Marie had chickened out at the last minute and was not there).

The room quickly filled up with about ninety people. I glanced at the clock. It was time to begin.

I got up in front of everyone, a bundle of nerves but trying my best to look sophisticated and composed. I thanked my husband, Ken, for incorporating The Beljanski Foundation, and my mother for accepting the position of President. Then I declared its first symposium officially open.

Surprisingly, from that nervous introduction on, everything went forward quite magically, especially considering my scarce knowledge of the science and zero experience in organizing a scientific symposium.

The doctors seemed to perfectly complement each other, as they addressed various topics and questioned each other in spontaneous and healthy mini-debates.

Dr. de Kuyper's presentation was highly anticipated, since this would be the first time he was going to speak publicly since the passing of his famous patient, President Mitterrand. Although Dr. Gubler, Mitterrand's anesthetist and last official doctor, had already made public in his book "Le Grand Secret"[1] that Mitterrand had been taking Beljanski's products, Dr. de Kuyper always remained very discreet about his relationship with the President. He offered an excellent presentation about long-term prostate cancer care, while carefully avoiding dropping any names. He laid down an exhaustive treatment protocol that included many dietary recommendations, as well as the use of all of my father's extracts: *Pao pereira* and *Rauwolfia vomitoria* for cancer, a very unique and specific golden leaf *Ginkgo biloba* extract to support the healing process (after the surgery and during all the radiotherapy), and RNA fragments during chemotherapy.

Dr. de Kuyper received a long round of applause.

Then, Professor Shoshan took the floor and offered another incredible presentation, revealing an intimate and profound understanding of my father's thinking. He explained how one discovery had led Beljanski to another, although each discovery was so massive it could seem, at the outset, as a world in itself. The greatest, most promising discovery, in Shoshan's opinion, was related to RNA fragments.

Since that time, he and I have had many discussions, but this is in substance what he told the audience that day in New York:

"As the numbers of cancer cases are rising, the pharmaceutical companies have developed an industry called the Cancer Industry, selling a short menu of "treatments." Available options are: cutting (surgery), burning (radiotherapy) or poisoning (chemotherapy) the bad cells. The outcome of each one is notoriously poor, and they are, more often than not, offered as a combination. In addition to the poor outcome, most anticancer treatments have a secondary, but pronounced destructive effect on healthy cells, including blood cells.

"Leukocytes (the blood cells that are the core of our immune system) and platelets (the cells in the blood that allow for clotting and repair when a blood vessel is damaged) are highly sensitive to chemotherapy, and resist it poorly. Quite often, during a cycle of chemotherapy treatments, the number of white blood cells drops dangerously, leaving the way open to infection, while the reduction in the number of platelets leads to hemorrhages. Chemotherapy must be halted periodically to allow time for the organs responsible for blood formation to recuperate; these arrests in treatment lower its effectiveness.

"Pharmaceutical companies have come up with some solutions based on growth factors to impede this drop in the number of platelets and white blood cells, but these products are so toxic that they cannot be taken for a long time, and certainly do not justify the hopes that they raised.

"Thinking first on analyzing how our body is naturally producing those precious cells, which are the core of our immune system, Beljanski thought of testing different RNA fragments in the presence of DNA. Why did he do this? A Japanese scientist had demonstrated that RNA fragments are essential for DNA synthesis (the first step of cell division).[2] Beljanski considered that these RNA fragments, called primers, might be more than a simple requirement for DNA replication; they might serve as a trigger. He had the intuition that the addition of primers to bone marrow cells could trigger DNA synthesis of those cells and the subsequent production of white blood cells and platelets.

"Beljanski isolated RNA fragments from the bone marrow and spleen of mammals, that is, from those parts of the organism where white blood cells and platelets are produced. Beljanski and his collaborators were hoping to discover which primers might enhance the multiplication of leukocytes and platelet cells. They succeeded. Once they understood the characteristics of the primers, Beljanski and his team could prepare them in quantity from a natural source: the RNA fragments were made from E. coli K-12 (a bacteria naturally present in the gut that does not cause sickness and does not promote mutations). Beljanski found these E. coli K-12 RNA fragments behaved as selective primers that stimulate the initiation of DNA synthesis in cells of the bone marrow yielding new white blood cells and new platelets, without side effects.[3]

"Beljanski went on to demonstrate that the new RNA fragments had no effect on the replication of DNA in cancerous tissue, even leukemic cells.[4] The next big question was whether those RNA fragments could be used to increase the numbers of white blood cells and platelets that had been depleted by radiotherapy or chemotherapy.

"In-depth experimentation was carried out on animals. Healthy rabbits were first given doses of a chemotherapy drug (anti-mitotic), whose effect on blood cells could be fatal to the animals. The experimenters chose products frequently used on humans: Endoxan (75 percent cyclophosphamide) because it is especially dangerous to white blood cells, and Daunorubucin, particularly harmful to platelets.[5]

"Rabbits received daily intravenous injections of Endoxan, each dose being forty times greater, proportionally in terms of weight, than the dose normally taken by a human in the course of one week, causing a drop of white blood cells expected to induce death of the animal within ten days.

"Then, RNA fragments were administered. The leukocyte count rose, and within twenty-four to forty-eight hours was normal again. Once the experiment was finished, the rabbits continued in good health, despite having received antimitotic doses far beyond the doses given in human therapy. Follow-up studies conducted one to two years after the experiment showed no side effects in the rabbits.

"The team also observed that in a healthy rabbit, the two main categories of white blood cells (polynuclears, the blood cells largely responsible for microbe defenses and lymphocytes, which are the main type of cell found in lymph) were present in more or less equal proportions. But one week of Endoxan creates a big unbalance between polynuclears and lymphocytes. That is, until the RNA fragments reestablished within 4 or 5 hours the normal equilibrium. The effect lasted for several days, and equilibrium was thereafter easily maintained by administering the same doses of RNA fragments at regular intervals.[6]

"To study the effects of RNA fragments on platelets, the number of platelets were reduced by means of Daunorobicin, administered in quantities once again much greater proportionally than those used in human medicine. Intravenous injections of 1.5mg/kg of Daunorobicin were given to rabbits for four consecutive days, leading to a drop in the platelet counts, which would mean the death of the animal by hemorrhage within six to eight days. But the RNA fragments brought the number of platelets back to its normal value within five to six days, and the animal lived. Repeated doses of RNA fragments did not lead to intolerance among rabbits treated with antimitotics, nor did they do so among the control group."[7]

"The discovery of Beljanski's RNA fragments was announced on June 5, 1978 by Professor Lepine at the Académie des Sciences and on the following day at the Académie de Médecine, as a non-toxic naturally originating product, not only able to re-establish normal white blood cell and platelet levels, but also to restore the leukocyte differential to equilibrium.[6]

"Beljanski's RNA fragments," continued professor Shoshan, "are natural oligoribonucleotides. These are small fragments of building blocks in a cell. The RNA fragments offered, for the first time, a means not only of maintaining normal white blood cell or platelet levels during radiotherapy or chemotherapy, but also of preserving normal ratios among the various kinds of white blood cells, notably those that fight infection. And that makes them, in my view, far superior to the manufactured granulocyte colony-stimulating factor (G-CSF) that is currently given to maintain white blood cells in those undergoing chemotherapy.

Professor Shoshan concluded: "G-CSF may be considered the gold standard, but the possibility that it acts as a growth factor for any tumor type, including myeloid (related to bone marrow), malignancies, and myelodysplasia (a disorder where the bone marrow does not produce enough healthy blood cells), cannot be excluded. Their safety in chronic myeloid leukemia and myelodysplasia has not been established. Worse, the safety and efficacy of G-CSF, when given simultaneously with cytotoxic chemotherapy, have not been established."

After the long round of applause receded, a doctor from Belgium intervened to present results showing that children treated with Beljanski's RNA fragments to stimulate their immune defenses clearly improved their psychological equilibrium and their scholastic performance (Yet another bombshell! There were so many, I was losing count).

She noted that European children were becoming more "Americanized" in their lifestyle. They eat more and more sugar (a "Western" diet), drink soda, and spend many sedentary hours in front of the television. These unhealthy habits greatly contribute to their weight gain. Obesity in children is becoming more of a problem, as is the rise in behavioral disorders. She was thrilled to report that children under her watch who were too agitated and incapable of focusing their attention became much calmer and showed clear progression in their studies, after taking RNA fragments sublingually once a week for several weeks.

About thirty participants immediately raised their hands to ask questions, and a high-level discussion followed.

"This is so exciting!" Dr. Schachter exclaimed, turning to me in awe, "And so original! I have never heard of anything like that before! And you said that there will be more tomorrow?"

His eyes were sparkling. I was so pleased!

But then, a doctor from Luxembourg shared that a company in Europe was producing RNA fragments made from baker's yeast selling them as Beljanski's product.

My stomach churned! *What??? Using my father's name?*

"The problem is that they do not seem to work so well," added the doctor. "I do not know if it is because of the yeast, or what, but I do not have the same results at all with those new ones."

I was floored. A company was usurping my father's reputation, taking advantage of his good name, and selling crap to sick people! This was clearly fraudulent activity. I immediately envisioned a flood of junk named "Beljanski" on the market, causing irreparable harm to my father's legacy.

My head was spinning. I could not wait for the end of the day to have some quiet time to think of the best action to take in response.

Over dinner, I couldn't speak of anything else.

"You want to sue them in Europe?" asked Ken. "Good luck with that. It will take you several years, and you will never be able to control or enforce anything."

I knew he was right.

We went to bed, exhausted from the activities of the day, but I could not sleep. I just lay staring up in the dark, as if the answer to this new dilemma I was facing would somehow magically drop down from the ceiling. The pinching in my stomach continued, more intense with each passing hour. Just when I thought I could not lie still in bed one moment longer, an idea suddenly dropped into my head. I bolted up, startled.

Trademark!

A myriad of thoughts assailed my mind at once.

What if they have already trademarked the Beljanski name? Then even I couldn't use it anymore, my father's name, my own name, without infringing on their rights! And what about the Foundation's name that I had just incorporated? Would I have to change the name? Why didn't I think of trademarking the name earlier? How could I have missed that? This is a miserable failure ... my miserable failure!

And then a hopeful thought transcended all the negative vibes.

Maybe they did not think of it either! Maybe there is still time for me to protect the Beljanski name!

I was out of bed and at the computer in a flash. Taking a deep breath, I tried to remain calm. Why was that machine always so slow when I was in a hurry?

Finally, the screen lit up bright in the dark room and I searched for "European Trademark Office" and then "Beljanski" trademark.

"What are you doing? Are you coming back to bed?" Ken's voice drifted in from the bedroom.

"Coming," I called, my mind totally occupied with the mission at hand. "Do you think they thought of trademarking the name?"

"Trademark?! Now?! At 2:00 a.m.?! When is this craziness going to end?!"

The voice was now indignant.

My fingers were running on the keyboard. This was important. Couldn't he understand?

I searched every possible combination of words and characters and ... Beljanski did not show up.

What a relief!

Still, I knew it did not mean that the name was available for sure. It could have been registered up to six months earlier without showing up yet in the database. I would have to learn to live with the anxiety for several months. But if the name had not been registered yet, perhaps I could...

"Sleep," I called out again. "I'll be back to bed soon."

I flipped on the desk lamp, pulled out my credit card, and proceeded with the registration without any further delay. I repeated the same procedure with the U.S. Patent and Trademark Office. Mission accomplished!

With a sigh of relief, I shut down the computer, turned off the desk lamp and crept back to bed.

Ken was sound asleep.

I rose from bed early despite my middle-of-the night Internet excursion. It was the second day of the seminar, and I began it with a little more confidence, knowing that I had taken care of a pressing issue that could have put a terrible damper on the meeting.

Professor Shoshan showed up early and pulled me aside.

"I could not sleep," he confided. "I have been thinking of those fake RNA fragments all night."

"Me too," I said. I told him how I had registered the trademark during the night.

He smiled. "You are thinking like a lawyer, but I am thinking like a scientist. Why are their RNAs not working? Once the RNA is purified and fragmented, should it not be sufficient? How could the source be so essential to the result?"

"I do not know much about science," I replied, "but any French woman who cooks a little bit—and we all do—will tell you that if you change the ingredients of a stew, you will change the result, hence the taste. That's why we value our family recipes."

"I get that. But it would make a very interesting research program."

I nodded.

Dr. Schachter arrived soon after, waving a notebook. "I came prepared this morning," he declared excitedly, "This is great."

The second day of the symposium was dedicated to hearing testimonials from the patients of many of the doctors who had lectured the first day. I was struck by the generosity of all those people who traveled for miles just to share how they had been helped, carried by the hope that their selfless effort would help others.

"How many pills? "How many times a day?" Dr. Schachter was asking each one, carefully noting every answer.

"All of this information is included in Dr. Marcowith's notebook that I gave you yesterday,"* Gérard whispered in my ear.

Oh, Great! I thought. *Now, I am the guardian of a knowledge treasure!*

Soon, it was time to part, and we all did so with great reluctance. Those two days had bonded us in a way that was quite remarkable. We now shared a common thread—a unique understanding of something profound that was about to happen.

---

*   See Bonus 1: Notes from Christian Marcowith, M.D.

We all promised to stay in touch. Professor Shoshan, however, was not going to leave without getting back to his research program idea.

"I do not have any of the E. coli based RNA fragments product," I protested. "This is the *one* I have not received."

I could see the professor was not going to take "no" for an answer.

"We could study the toxicity and effectiveness of the growth factors which are currently given to people, along with chemotherapy, as a baseline, and that would lay the road for studying your RNA fragments later," he said urgently. "Once you are able to get them manufactured, we will compare the two and show the world that the RNA fragments are a far better option."

I wasn't convinced. "I have no idea how to get that product re-manufactured, since everything was destroyed or seized in the lab," I said. "Frankly, I am not sure that this whole thing is for me. I am a lawyer, not a business person."

"What do you think is more important?" he asked shrewdly. His blue piercing eyes were gazing intensely at me, and he managed to be intimidating despite his small, frail figure.

"What good is it to win a lawsuit if your immune system is down the drain? Those RNA fragments are not only for people undergoing chemotherapy, but are for everybody whose immune system is down. The immune system is the cornerstone of good health. There is an Arab proverb: 'He who has health has hope, and he who has hope has everything.' You have the power to give everything to the world, and I will help you with the studies to document it."

I searched for a polite but sufficiently evasive answer to protect the frontal assault on my legal career.

"For starters, I have no power at all. But are you telling me that the fight before the European Court of Human Rights is not important? (At the time, *Beljanski vs. France* was still in full swing as I battled the French government in The European Court of Human Rights.) That organizing this symposium is not important? Creating a foundation to carry on my father's work is not important? I am defending my father's honor and spreading the word about his work. I think it is the most important task I could do right now."

Just then Gérard came in, eager to join the conversation.

I was hoping he would provide a welcome distraction, but instead Gérard put his right hand on his heart, bent over as if he was saluting a Japanese dignitary, and declared, "Professor, this is the happiest day of my life. Yes! Let's do this!" Turning to tease me, he added, "I think I know somebody who could help."

This whole "promised mission" was turning out to be a bit more than I had bargained for. And now to pursue a research project? Should I recognize the foolishness of the adventure, or should I go for it, knowing full well that I did not know anything about the feasibility of my father's products, their science, or their distribution except that the French government did not want them around.

I couldn't even consider a business plan. But as I was contemplating the idea and naming it "the craziest idea ever," I found myself slowly warming up to it, and even to its pet name. I started going through the list of what we would need.

First, we would need funding. I immediately thought of selling the little apartment I still owned in Paris. I had inherited the apartment from my grandparents, and had kept it even after moving to New York. I cherished their memory so much that selling had not yet been an option. But now, I realized I was considering carrying on a legacy much larger than myself, than my own life. I was in service not just to my father, but to all those who needed my help.

I knew right away that this was going to be a full-time commitment. I would have to give up the legal career I had worked so hard for. That was a heart-rending realization. And then, what if I failed? The thought was terrifying, causing my stomach to twist into a giant knot.

But then again, what is failure? Is failure not trying? Could I ever be content with my life if I turned my back on all this love and all these expectations? I certainly would be a disappointment to everyone involved. And not only to them, but also to myself ... forever!

I decided that not trying seemed even worse than trying and not succeeding.

Although I was short one business plan, I at least had the beginnings of a plan of action—I called a broker in Paris to list my apartment.

I also reached for the papers that Gérard and my mother had left with me, the ones I never had a chance to look through during the symposium. I was vaguely hoping to find in them some providential guidance for what to do next.

Beside the Marcowith notebook, there was a several-page manuscript in my father's handwriting titled "The anticancer Agent PB-100, Selectively Active on Malignant Cells, Inhibits Multiplication of Sixteen Malignant Cell Lines, even Multidrug Resistant."[8]

I knew that "PB-100" was the code name used by my father for his *Pao pereira* extract. But what should I do with a manuscript?

I kept searching and, finally, in the envelope brought by my mother, I found a letter sent to my father from the scientific journal *Genetics and Molecular Biology*. The letter, about eight months old and signed by the editor-in-chief of the journal, was addressing my father as "Dear Referee," for evaluation of the merits of a scientific paper.

I didn't even know that my father had been a referee for scientific journals!

The first thing to do seemed obvious: be polite.

I called the journal, asked for the editor-in-chief, introduced myself, and explained that it was due to my father's passing that the editor had never received an answer to his letter. The editor expressed heart-felt condolences. He had, indeed, been surprised that his letter had remained unanswered. My father had been such a great contributor!

I heard myself say, "I have in my hands his last manuscript. Would you be interested in publishing it?"

"Send it to me," he replied. "If it is a good fit for our journal, it will be our honor to publish it."

I had the distinct intuition he would publish the manuscript. Now, with an upcoming publication on *Pao pereira* on the horizon, the next step was obvious.

I had to source the botanical.

CHAPTER FIVE
HUNTING FOR PAO PEREIRA

"Life is tough, my darling, but so are you."

STEPHANIE BENNET-HENRY

M any times, we would not move forward if we knew what lay ahead of us. Life is filled with teachable moments, and here I learned that it is easy to make a vow, but not quite so easy to carry it out....

The barrels I received from Bernard Fourche only contained about a six-month supply of the valuable plant extracts. If I were to create and establish a foundation that would carry on my father's work and research, I would need a lot more product than that. I had to find many kilograms—maybe even a ton—of the *Pao pereira* bark. And fast.

Originally, my father worked with samples provided by the Pasteur Institute in French Guiana. Founded in 1940, this offspring of the Paris Pasteur Institute has helped researchers access numerous tropical botanicals. When the need arose, and larger quantities of the botanicals were required, my father met with an Air France flight attendant who knew of a coffee grower in Cayenne, French Guiana, who was able to share with my father where to find the *Pao pereira* bark.

I searched all available listings of coffee growers, searched for ocean freight records, wrote to the president of the local Chamber of Commerce asking for clues, and, eventually, was able to locate the coffee grower's son, only to learn from the son that his father had recently passed away and he did not know much about his father's business.

It seemed a fruitless journey, and I had no idea where else to turn for help.

How did my father identify this extract? I wondered. *Just randomly screening hundreds of extracts through his Oncotest?*

I learned from a medical journalist, Claudy Nordau[1], that the first potent anticancer extract that Beljanski had identified was not the *Pao pereira* extract, as I had assumed, but a very specific extract from *Rauwolfia vomitoria*. And *Rauwolfia* had come to my father's attention because it was part of a large controversy.

Rauwolfia serpentina (and to a certain extent, its close cousin *Rauwolfia vomitoria*) is an erect, tropical, evergreen sub-shrub. Known as "Sarpagandha," it has been used for millennia in India as one of the very important Ayurvedic herbs. The paste of its roots, mixed with rose water, is said to ameliorate mental stress, headache, giddiness, and to induce sound sleep. It was even reported that Mahatma Gandhi used it without reservation as a tranquilizer during his lifetime.[2]

In the early 1950s, Jacques Servier was a young a French doctor and businessman looking to launch his own pharmaceutical company. Servier was interested in the new and lucrative hypertension market. He dedicated his PhD thesis to the study of the Indian plant *Rauwolfia serpentina*[3], but knew that he was never going to become rich with an herb. (Yes, this is the very same Servier who would lend his name to the Laboratoire Servier and launch a drug called "mediator" which contained dexfenfluramine. Servier would later be charged in 2009 in France for consumer fraud, manslaughter, and defrauding the French healthcare system.[4] Dexfenfluramine would also eventually be pulled from the U.S. market by the FDA because it was deemed too dangerous).

In the pharmaceutical industry, one has to get a patent in order to make big money. To be patentable, something must be new. Therefore, the pharmaceutical industry always has to "twist" nature in order to create a new patentable invention. The problem for Jacques Servier is that there was nothing new—and, therefore, nothing patentable—with an herb that had been used for millennia in India. Hence, the "twist": rather than using the plant itself, as used in traditional medicine, he would create a patentable product by using a plant extract.

In 1955, Servier Laboratories launched "Sarpagan," a Rauwolfia extract sold as a drug to treat hypertension. Sarpagan would be a standardized extract containing a fixed and large quantity of the main alkaloid present in the plant, known as reserpine. Reserpine was supposed to be the active agent able to fight hypertension, with some of the other alkaloids naturally present in the plant playing a less important role.*

Servier was right about the hypertension market: the availability of medications to reduce blood pressure has dramatically changed the impact and natural course of its treatment. It had transformed the role of physicians in society, creating an unprecedented windfall for doctors and the pharmaceutical industry.

As once written by Dr. Ronald C. Hamdy, editor-in-chief of the *Southern Medical Journal*: "Before these medications were available, patients went to see their doctors only if they were not feeling well or were sick. Once these medications became available, asymptomatic and otherwise healthy people went to see their doctors to find out if they were healthy. Doctors were now needed to reassure people that they were healthy, because feeling healthy was no longer synonymous with being healthy [...] It is still debated whether Roosevelt's hypertension and probable complicating heart failure clouded his judgment during the Yalta Conference with Churchill and Stalin, only eight weeks before his death. How different would the world have been after the Second World War II had the United States, Britain and France liberated Berlin as opposed to the Soviet Union? Similarly, one may wonder what would have happened if Stalin, who also had hypertension, did not sustain a fatal stroke in 1953 and was still alive and in control of the Soviet Union during the Cuban missile crisis."[5]

Doctors began to routinely prescribe the reserpine–based hypertension medicine. According to a report produced by U.S. National Institutes of

---

* A standardized herbal extract is an herb extract that has one or more components present in a specific, guaranteed amount, and the others get eliminated. The intention behind the standardization of herbs is to guarantee that the consumer is getting a product which is consistent from batch to batch. However, plants in their natural state contain a complex blend of phytochemicals, and the full medicinal value of herbs is most likely due to their internal complexity and to the interactions of the different components within the body rather than to one of its specific components. Moreover, the fact that a whole plant has been safely used for centuries does not guarantee that a selective and concentrated extract will be safe.

Health (NIH) in 1976, the volume of reserpine sold in the U.S. alone was 440,000 lbs.[6] However, they soon started to wonder about a possible serious side effect: could the hypertensive drug be carcinogenic?[7]

An alarming number of women taking the reserpine-based hypertension medicine had been shown to develop breast cancer. Several studies were funded with confusing results: a 1984 study suggested that *Rauwolfia* alkaloids did not increase the risk of breast cancer,[8] while a 1985 study suggested that women exposed to long-term *Rauwolfia* use had an elevated risk of developing breast cancer.[9]

The controversy was raging in medical circles.

Dr. Jean Bugiel, a family doctor practicing in Paris, had been my grandparents' doctor for decades.

One day, my grandmother had a serious case of the flu, and called for Dr. Bugiel. He responded quickly, showing up at our doorstep in record time.

My father just so happened to be around that day, and the doctor and the scientist immediately headed off in private consultation, almost forgetting about my bedridden grandmother and her flu. The controversy surrounding Servier's *Rauwolfia* extract quickly came up in the conversation between the good doctor and the visionary scientist.

After that conversation, my father decided to test Servier's Sarpagan with his Oncotest and made the following discovery: Sarpagan essentially contained two active alkaloids—reserpine, the main one, was highly cytotoxic and carcinogenic, while alstonine, the secondary alkaloid, exhibited valuable anticarcinogenic properties. Beljanski separated the two, discarded the reserpine, and kept only the good one—the alstonine.

Thus, Beljanski's specific *Rauwolfia* extract is devoid of reserpine and rich in alstonine. It is gentle on normal cells, does not exhibit any of the anticipated toxic side effects generally associated with reserpine, and is selectively effective on cancerous cells. This specific extract doesn't do much for hypertension. Its beauty is that it seems to "know" that it must go to cancerous cells, just like the molecules used by the body for the regulation of its physiology "know" where to go to fight cancerous cells.[10]

This very specific and selective activity, which spares normal cells, represented an important departure from conventional cancer treatments, which are brutal and blind, and work aggressively on both cancer cells and healthy cells.

Beljanski couldn't wait to announce to Mr. Servier that his Sarpagan contained two very different alkaloids, including one that could distinguish between cancer cells and healthy cells and selectively suppress the former ones. But when Beljanski told him, Servier was not interested in learning Sarpagan's faults.

Servier's answer was immediate, and definitive: "There is no difference between normal cells and cancer cells." Greedy Jacques Servier bypassed the opportunity to develop the first specific anticancer drug.

In 1955, after the discovery of the polio vaccine, President Eisenhower predicted that "In twenty years, cancer will be defeated." The U.S. started to pour money into anticancer research soon thereafter. Indeed, the fight to defeat cancer took a decisive turn within twenty years, since it was in December 1975 that Beljanski introduced his first cancer drug to Jacques Servier. What President Eisenhower had not foreseen, however, was that the conquering of cancer would not happen in the U.S., and that the discovery would go unacknowledged.

Purifying *Rauwolfia* is a messy and expensive operation. Beljanski turned to his books on chemistry to see if other plants had molecules similar to alstonine. There he found the perfect candidate on paper, flavopereirine, smaller than alstonine, with the similar characteristic of one positively and one negatively charged nitrogen, readily available from the bark of the *Pao pereira* tree.

With purification and quality control so vital to the production of Beljanski's *Rauwolfia* extract, yet so difficult, finding a way to locate an ample supply of *Pao pereira* was paramount for me to continue his legacy.

Just when I was feeling a little hopeless and quite helpless about the whole matter, I received a wonderful surprise—a phone call from the coffee grower's son!

He told me about a woman in Brazil who might know how to find the *Pao pereira*. Her business was exporting hearts of palms, he explained, and she was very familiar with the rainforest. I felt I had nothing to lose and much to gain, so I decided to go to Brazil to meet with this "Heart of Palm Lady."

My first stop was Rio de Janeiro, and its botanical garden, which has two specimens of the sought-after tree. Armed with a map of the botanical garden, I found their *Pao pereira* trees, and thoroughly examined them, taking many pictures. I noticed that the trunks were abundantly shedding, and that the soil surrounding each tree was covered with little pieces of bark. Intuitively, I reached for a Kleenex and collected as many flecks as my handkerchief could hold. I touched, smelled, and even tried to chew the pieces of bark, but it was so very bitter that I had to spit it right back.

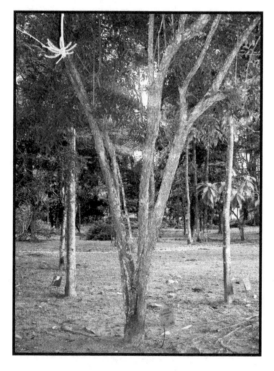

Specimen of Pao pereira at the Botanical Garden in Rio de Janeiro, Brazil (Photograph: Sylvie Beljanski, 2001. © The Beljanski Foundation, Inc.)

After visiting the trees, I went to the botanical garden's public library and checked out every book available on the *Pao pereira* tree.

Geissospermum vellosii, or *Geissospermum leave velloso*, also known as *Pau pereira* or *Pao pereira,* is a common tree native to many countries in South America. Used in traditional medicine for centuries, is also very much a part of South American popular culture. The first official monograph on the benefits of *Pao pereira* goes back to 1848, when Ezequiel Correa Dos Santos presented his thesis "*Monographia do Geissospermum vellosii vulgo Pao pereira*" to the Faculty of Medicine of Rio de Janeiro.[11] *Pao pereira*'s traditional use is well-recognized as an excellent tonic and powerful remedy against intermittent fevers.

Most interesting for me to learn was that the bark sheds naturally all year round, making its collection perfectly sustainable.

At this point, I was looking forward to meeting the Heart of Palm Lady. I connected with her by phone, and was amazed at her knowledge of the plant world. She was indeed familiar with *Pao pereira*, and knew where we could find it. She invited me to join her in the city of Manaus.

A vibrant industrial city of two million people located in the heart of the Amazon rainforest, Manaus is rich with nineteenth century architecture, recalling a time when rubber made it the richest city in South America. I had no time for sightseeing, however. My Heart of Palm Lady, a short and authoritative woman of indigenous Indios heritage, made a few phone calls, and before I knew it, we were embarking on a voyage to find the prized *Pao pereira* tree.

We planned to travel upstream on the Rio Negro river, a tributary to the Amazon, and then go deep into the jungle by foot. Eventually we would reach an Indios settlement where I would be introduced to the head of the local tribe. A small backpack with the barest necessities (including my camera, a ceremonial present for the tribe, and a bottle of water) was all I could carry.

So there I was on that sizzling hot day, cramped with three other people—the Heart of Palm Lady with her broken English, and two men who only spoke Portuguese—on an elongated, narrow motor boat, chugging along through the murky darkness of the Rio Negro (The jet-black color of the water, reason for the river's name, is caused by the decomposition of phenol-containing vegetation from swamps—yuck!).

Although communication was difficult, I understood I was not to shift my weight to the right or left at any time because the boat just might tip over. There were no crocodiles to worry about on this river, but I had to be careful of the piranhas. *How comforting?* I shivered despite the heat, and sat as straight and still as possible as we chugged along under the hot Amazon sun.

Hours passed. We could not go any faster against the powerful flow of the river. My legs were cramped and my back felt as though it had been starched straight. How I longed to get out and have a good stretch. Well, I always heard that you should be careful with wishes, because they just might come true. As we finally neared the bank of the river, the man that was directing the boat tried to gently turn so we could get ashore more easily, but turning a canoe on such a powerful torrent was not an easy task, and *smack,* we were all in the murky waters of this not-so-majestic river.

The boat had capsized!

Without thinking, I found myself fervently paddling with one arm, while desperately trying to keep my camera above my head with the other.

Thankfully we all reached the bank of the river and crawled onto the gritty, hot sand, exhausted and soaking wet. But there was no resting or taking time to recover. We had to get to the village before sundown. As I had no change of clothes or extra shoes, I trudged on, silent. I did not feel good at all, but then again, I was on a mission. I had goals to fulfill and promises to keep.

I sighed and kept walking.

Brazil is an extremely important agricultural and industrial country, with the strongest economy in Latin America. It is the world's largest coffee and sugarcane producer, and the second-largest soybean producer. Despite all those riches, however, extreme poverty is still widespread in many parts of the country.

When we finally arrived at the village in the jungle, children ran out to greet us—beautiful, smiling children with dirty faces, tattered clothes, and bare feet. There was no electricity or running water, and our wet jackets were hung up to dry on a frazzled rope stretched across two weathered wooden poles. We were ushered into a dilapidated, two-room hut with an earthen floor.

It had been arranged for us to spend the night at the home of a local family, so I did not expect fancy amenities by any means. But even with my already low expectations, I can say it was still a bit of a culture shock to see the meager living conditions in this tiny, indigenous village. They seemed happy, nonetheless, and very excited to host us. I watched, a little leery, as they rushed about preparing supper, which was a local delicacy —boiled river snake. I had never eaten boiled snake before, but I was hungry and open to trying new things. However, after that meal I knew for a fact that I did not like boiled snake. It was slimy and chewy, although it had been boiling for hours, and had a very distinctive taste that I can only describe as extremely disgusting.

There was no bathroom in this tiny village, and I did not even inquire as to how one was supposed to take care of nature's call. I put my mind to other things, like my still-soaked clothing.

We conversed as best we could for a while around the flickering candlelight as the shadows of the night closed in around us. Then we were shown to an empty room, which contained our beds: hammocks hanging from the ceiling. (Hammock sleeping is a means of protection from foraging nocturnal animals). I hesitated to leave my still wet shoes on the floor, since I feared they would become home to insects during the night, so I kept them on and climbed up into my hammock.

As I laid in the hammock, I thought again about my desire to answer nature's call. The real challenge would be finding my way out of the hut, and venturing out in the dark, vast Amazon forest. The thought was not exactly appealing at the moment, but I later learned that such an experience was actually quite humbling and unique. To find yourself joining the animals out in the noisy Amazon forest, you really understand that you are not alone in the universe. And you certainly are not as high and mighty as you thought you were. You realize you are just a microscopic being in the middle of a great and very occupied vastness.

The sun rose early the next morning, signaling all that it was time to wake up. I arose with my clothes still wet, clammy, and clinging to my skin. Not a nice feeling.

I climbed down from my hammock and stretched. A large, hairy spider quickly scurried out of my way and I felt grateful I had kept my shoes on. Our host family served us coffee in dirty metallic cups around a wood-burning stove, and we set off on the next phase of our journey.

We needed to travel by foot through the Amazon rainforest to the next village, which was about five hours away. The uncomfortable feeling of wet and sticky was still there but as we walked and the sun grew hotter, my clothes and shoes eventually dried out. I was told that we were lucky it was the dry season, because that walk would be impossible during the rainy season. Since, in my ignorance I had not planned the trip around the seasons, I made a conscious effort to appreciate my luck and be grateful. I needed all the positive reinforcement that I could muster, as I was following those three strangers, including two men with axes, deep into the forest. I could have disappeared into that forest, and nothing I had in my possession would have saved me. Not my camera, nor my American Express card, and not even my cell phone. Relying on human connection was all I had. As we slowly progressed on the narrow path, I tried to make conversation despite the language barrier. I asked how we would properly identify the *Pao pereira* trees in the middle of all the luxurious vegetation surrounding us. And then, once the trees were identified, how would we transport the bark to the river?

Pointing at what looked like some old dung, they explained that the villagers had donkeys to carry everything back and forth, the river being their lifeline connection to the outside world. Some of the villagers even made routine trips to the city to sell Brazilian nuts, coconuts, and some handicrafts for tourists, and bring back food and wares for the use of the villagers. *Pao pereira* would benefit from that same donkey-to-boat "infrastructure."

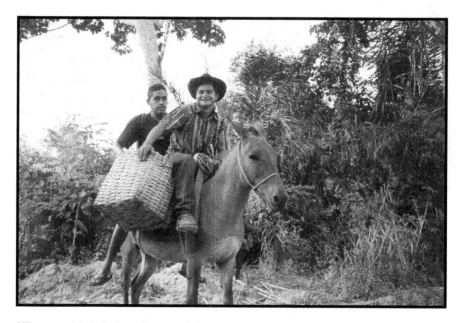

Villagers and their donkeys (Photograph Sylvie Beljanski, 2001.)

As we continued deeper into the forest, I was amazed at the vastness and majesty of the great rainforest. I stretched my neck and gazed up in awe at the massive trees that seemed to have no tops. I could not see the sky above the tremendous entanglement of branches and leaves. It was magnificent to behold and to hear. I couldn't distinguish between the varieties of noises, nor could I tell from where they all originated. It was as if a great invisible orchestra was rehearsing, directed by an unseen conductor. I felt like I was in a different universe.

Finally we arrived at the next village and were received with heartfelt excitement by the entire population.

I was "The American" representing for them another world completely—a civilization none of them had ever experienced.

One beautiful little girl ran up to me and touched my leg, as if to make sure I was real. Representing America was a little bit ironic since I myself felt like an immigrant (although technically I was born an American citizen), but I stood up straight and gave a broad smile, committed to making America proud.

Everyone was very friendly, and I began to wonder how the Beljanski Foundation's work could benefit them, as well.

Would purchasing orders of Pao pereira really give them something of value?

I couldn't think of what they would need that could be purchased with money. In a remote village without electricity, what would someone want to buy? Certainly not a TV or a refrigerator.

I was introduced to the chief of the village and the Heart of Palm Lady translated. I explained that I needed a sustainable production of the bark of *Pao pereira*. It was very important to me that the bark was obtained without harming the tree, in order to both preserve the environment and sustain the business opportunity. He confirmed that he would be able to provide large quantities of *Pao pereira* as it grew in abundance around the village. He showed me one of the trees. It seemed much larger and much taller than those I had seen in the botanical garden, but it had similar leaves and the bark was properly peeling away.

I chewed a little piece of it and immediately recognized the distinctive, extremely bitter taste.

I was delighted and asked what I could do for the village in return. Giving money to a community that did not even have a bank in which to deposit it made little sense. I knew I would have to go beyond money. I felt I carried the social opportunity, and going along with it, the social responsibility, to really touch the lives of those people. After some discussion, part English, part Portuguese, and mostly gesture, we agreed that the first things they would need would be an electric generator in the village, and also to build a school. I was elated. I felt like I was making history.

We concluded our conversation and the women prepared lunch, which was more of the local delicacy. I did not care for it at all, but as I did not want to offend my host, I proceeded to stuff my face with more boiled snake. When the ordeal of lunch was completed, we started the walk back to the river where the little boat was waiting. Walking back was more frightening than coming as it began to get dark, and the noises of the forest no longer seemed musically charming but rather alarming. And I was very much aware that I was at the mercy of those two men trudging before me on the narrow path with axes over their shoulders. Finally we reached the river and I saw the boat bobbing up and down on the water.

However, my relief was short-lived.

After climbing aboard the boat, we were assailed by an onslaught of mosquitoes. Can you imagine trying to shoo away mosquitoes without upsetting the boat? This time, we were going in the direction of the water, and it was like the torrent was carrying our little boat. The waters were very choppy, and the boat's engine had to work hard to keep us moving in the right direction. The strong smell of the engine's gas was choking and nauseating. I started to feel lightheaded and soon my stomach began to churn to the rhythm of the water. The combination of the mosquitoes, the smell of the gas, the choppy waters, and the snake that I could not digest was too much for me. I couldn't help myself. I became completely sick, and had no choice but to let go of the snake. Between my heaves, I could hear the men yelling.

"Don't bend! Don't bend! We are going to tip over again!"

Don't bend?!

I passed out.

How I got back to Manaus and to the hotel, I do not know. The next clear recollection I have is boarding the plane to Rio de Janeiro to catch my connection back to New York.

"Coffee? Guarana juice? Açaí juice?"

The flight attendant was gently leaning towards me, offering her local refreshments.

It suddenly hit me: all the choices the flight attendant offered were mass-market products whose ingredients were easily sourced in quantity. *Pao pereira* was never going to be one of them.

How many bags of bark could a donkey carry? How many trips to the river could a donkey perform during one dry season? I had to accept that this was never going to become a large-scale production.

And if it was going to remain forever small, how would I ever make enough money to meet all the quality control requirements to produce the extracts, finance the research, and get the word out?

I was anticipating coming home with a renewed appreciation for hot running water, electricity, a decent mattress, and other wonders that define modern comfort. But, I couldn't help wondering: what is the real price we pay for those luxuries?

"Everyone has the right to life, liberty and security of person," states Article Three of the Universal Declaration of Human Rights. My father's liberty and security, and then his right to live, were eventually taken away through the abuse of modern Western institutions. Is life much less safe in the unregulated jungles? Does the Western idea of "right to life" include the right to maintain life through universal access to healthcare? Does the security of the person include access to any medical treatment of one's choice? What if the preferred treatment includes a dietary supplement made from a tree bark available only in small quantities, where universal access is just physically impossible? Is it a luxury, or a right?

My mind was drifting....

At home, I found my answering machine blinking.

The first message was from *Genetics and Molecular Biology*. As I had anticipated, the editor-in-chief had kindly accepted my father's manuscript for publication, and his message informed me that the paper would appear in the following issue.[12]

The second message was from Professor Shoshan. Hadassa University had agreed to study the safety of granulocytes given in conjunction with chemotherapy to establish a baseline preceding a later study on the benefits of the RNA fragments. Before he could start with the research program, however, he needed his research department to purchase all the necessary laboratory equipment.

The third message was from Gérard Weidlich. A French judge had ordered the return of my father's laboratory equipment to CIRIS, but had also ordered its sale to pay for all the bills that had piled up since the French army had seized everything and put a halt to all activity. Gérard was seeking my advice.

Isn't it ironic? Could it be possible that Shoshan needs to buy what Gérard needs to sell?

The last message was from Michael Schachter. He was considering lecturing about my father's work at a conference organized by the American College for Advancement in Medicine (ACAM). Dedicated to educating physicians and other health care professionals on the safe and effective application of integrative medicine, this nonprofit organization includes approximately eight-hundred members. I froze with anxiety.

What if they all want the products?

Dr. Schachter added that he would not be able to present before another year because it was too late to submit for this year.

Ouf! Temporary relief!

However, he suggested that I join him with a booth the following week at this year's convention in Las Vegas.

I turned to Ken who so far had not seemed very interested in hearing about the Amazon.

"It looks like I have to create a booth for next week and fly to Las Vegas," I said.

"*Las Vegas!* Now, that's exciting! I'm going with you."

CHAPTER SIX
JACKPOT

"Luck is flow and force. There's no power that can fully take that into account; fate is still wavering."

Nobuyuki Fukumoto

When I returned Gérard Weidlich's call, I learned that my father's entire laboratory was for sale, with all its considerable lab equipment. Bernard Fourche had already made an offer with the Court-appointed receiver (Gérard had explained this to me from a phone booth, as he suspected his home phone line was being tapped.)

"Fourche thinks that if he can get all the machines and instruments, he can take them out of France—most likely to Belgium or Germany—because it is too dangerous to do anything here in France. But once he has everything, he plans to start quickly with production, at least of the RNA fragments. He claims that he has befriended the head of the bacteriology department at some local university who is willing to provide him with enough E. coli k-12 bacteria* to start manufacturing the RNA fragment product. Also, he says that he will need, at least in the beginning, your mother's help to learn the technology."

---

* E. coli k-12 is known to be very safe, non-pathogenic bacteria, often used in molecular biology as both a tool and a model organism. And because bacteria can be grown in quantity, the product has no manufacturing limit.

I was grateful for Bernard Fourche courageously stepping up, but I had mixed feelings about letting go of my father's entire laboratory.

On the other hand, what could I possibly do with an entire state-of-the-art, scientific laboratory?

"Did you get an inventory? How much was Fourche's offer?" I asked Gérard. Unfortunately, he had not been given any more details.

I just have to learn to let it go....

Dr. Schachter's last message about Las Vegas sounded most promising. I booked a flight for my husband, Ken, and me, and looked forward to those few travel hours to Las Vegas. It would be my first opportunity to share with him everything that happened in Brazil and pick his brain regarding the sale of the laboratory.

As I was relating my story, Ken sat there rolling his eyes and shaking his head. Finally, he exploded: "There was no need to offer to build a school! Do you have any idea how much this is going to cost? How can you commit to something when you don't even have an estimate? I am sure that a donation of old books or a payment towards the salary of a part-time teacher would have been good enough!"

That wasn't the reaction I was hoping for.

Maybe I had gotten a little bit ahead of myself....

"As for your father's lab," Ken continued, "it's probably not worth more than the scrap of the metal of the machines. Frankly, I do not understand you. I see that you are possessed with this crazy story, but if you have to start looking for trees, why on earth do you have to start immediately looking for the one most difficult to locate? Why don't you focus on something easy, like the one Dr. de Kuyper mentioned at the symposium? The *Ginkgo biloba*? At least this tree is everywhere, even growing in New York streets. You can stay here and hug them to your content! No need for silly, expensive trips around the world and getting involved in the school building business!"

Heart and head do not always work well together.

I was about to explain that my father's *Ginkgo* extract was exclusively made from golden leaves—these leaves turn yellow only once a year for one month or so before they fall off the tree and securing hundreds of kilograms of them during that one month each year could prove to be another tricky task. Suddenly a memory flashed back to me.

I was looking forward to turning sixteen. Perhaps it would bring with it boldness, excitement, and maybe even romance.

I was a straight-A student in one of the best high schools in Paris, but that did nothing to help me overcome my extreme shyness and gave me zero experience in the social life department. Certainly becoming "older" would make a difference.

I didn't have to wait until the anticipated birthday. A school project that included a review of a theater play was the perfect opportunity for inviting home my secret little crush. The plan was to leave school together, stop by my place for dinner, and then go to the theater. The thought of the whole matter's potential gave me goosebumps. Could this be considered a date?

We left the school laughing as my (dare I say it) "date's" suave outgoing personality had helped pull me out of my shell. Everything was going so well— until the moment I pushed open the front door of my parents' apartment.

The floor was covered with a pile of golden Ginkgo leaves, several inches thick. They were spread all over the rooms like a huge, smelly, wall-to-wall, botanical carpet! I was appalled. How would I ever live this down? No way could I ever pretend at school to be a cool popular girl! Gone was any hope of puppy love! Ginkgo had made me a freak!

"That's the best way to get them dry!" my father's deep, burly voice intoned as he met us at the door. My mother was nodding emphatically in agreement. It was clear that my parents were as insensitive to the epic proportions of my teenage angst as I was to their reason for carpeting our home with tree leaves.

I smiled at the memory.

Should I ask my husband how he feels about a plush carpet of Ginkgo leaves drying on the dining room floor?

I decided against testing his sense of humor.

I chose instead to sit back and close my eyes, and as I did, my mind began to drift into contemplation of the golden *Ginkgo's* unique properties, and how my family got involved with the collection of tree leaves.

It was April 26, 1986, and the Chernobyl nuclear power plant in Ukraine had suffered the worst catastrophic failure in the history of the nuclear industry. As reported by the United Nations Scientific Committee on the Effects of Atomic Radiation, the complete meltdown of the reactor core, followed by the ten-day free emission of radionuclides into the atmosphere, caused the deaths (within a few painful days or weeks) of thirty power plant employees and firemen (and twenty-eight more with acute radiation syndrome). The accident caused the evacuation of thousands of people from Belarus, the Russian Federation, and Ukraine. Vast territories of those three countries (at that time republics of the Soviet Union) were contaminated, and trace deposits of released radionuclides was measurable in all countries of the northern hemisphere.[1]

With the Cold War still in full swing, the identification of an effective agent following radiation exposure immediately became a major priority, not only in radiological medicine, but also for the U.S. military. By 1987, the Pentagon had come up with ethylsulphanyl phosphonic acid, or ethiotos, also known as WR-2721. Unfortunately, WR-2721 not only had to be kept refrigerated and administered intravenously, but it also produced nausea, vomiting, diarrhea, and hypotension.[2] Despite those severe flaws, the U.S. Army decided to keep funding the investigation of this compound through contracts with its various western allies. The French Army was one of them, and soon looked to sub-contract with laboratories willing to work with radiation. This led them to Mirko Beljanski, who was interested in accessing radiation, not only to test WR-2721, but also to see how his own products reacted.

Beljanski had become very interested in *Ginkgo biloba* after learning that six trees growing one to two kilometers from the 1945 atom bomb explosion of Hiroshima had survived the blast.[3] Beljanski had noticed that in the plasma of cancer patients specific enzymes called ribonucleases* (RNase) extensively degrade RNAs. After further research, he went on to create a preparation based on the golden leaves (when leaves age they turn yellow and synthesize different profiles of molecules) of the *Ginkgo biloba* tree, which he found to be capable of efficiently regulating the in vitro and in vivo RNase activity.

---

* Since then, many studies have expanded their focus not only on changes occurring in these enzymes during the cancer process but also on those changes induced by radiations. Nowadays, RNase is even considered a cancer marker by several authors.

Taken during and after exposure to radiation this specific golden leaf extract of *Ginkgo biloba* protects, prevents, and even reverses (which to some means "heals") the fibrosis caused by excessive radiation, and brings patients' plasma RNase activity back to normal. In my father's laboratory the extract turned out to do just as well as WR-2721, without the side effects. Beljanski published his results,[4] but by then the Berlin Wall had fallen and military officials had lost interest in the subject.

Nevertheless, several French doctors were quick to see the benefit of a product that supported the healing process after surgery and helped protect against radiation-induced skin fibrosis.

They started to ask for it.

My maternal grandfather, Pr. René Lucas, was a distinguished scholar, a member of the prestigious *Academie des Sciences*, and recently retired from his position of Director of the Paris School of Physics and Chemistry as well as Professor of Physics at the Sorbonne. He took it upon himself to scour the city's municipal parks with a backpack and collect as many leaves as he could in season. My grandmother tagged along, and together they were a very effective pair—until they were caught for stealing leaves!

But in the meantime, the golden *Ginkgo* extract had already benefitted thousands of people.

My musings were cut short as we landed in Las Vegas.

After emerging from a week in the Amazon rainforest, Las Vegas appeared to me as the surreal antithesis of all things natural. The convention was held at Caesars Palace—a sprawling Roman-themed venue, adorned with fake atrium, fake coliseum, fake fountains, columns and statues everywhere. Inside the "palace," aisles as wide as streets were lined with slot machines, along with shops that blared deafening music and flashed blinking, blinding lights. I couldn't help but compare this unmelodious clamor to the majestic natural symphony I had recently experienced in the Amazon.

We checked in and headed upstairs to quickly freshen up.

I didn't take long. I was eager to reach the convention floor and set up our booth, which I had ordered online.

The booth had been shipped in a large box that was waiting for me at the hotel reception desk. And so was a big headache. The booth had looked good online, classy and easy to set up. In reality, it proved to be a complicated, Lego-like contraption.

Ken, having little patience for any DIY assembling project, declared that he would check how the other booths were coping, and promptly left. I stuck with the challenge. It took me about an hour to finally put it together somewhat. It was the best I could do for the time being, so I left it as it was and went to find Ken.

I slowly traversed the immense room, peering right and left at the booths, lined up in long alleys in alphabetical order. Hundreds of exhibitors had come to this conference, and it was amazing to see how diverse in sizes and looks their booths were.

Integrative medicine is a really diverse industry.

Since the late 1990s, the lure of catering to the needs of an aging population crippled with increasing rates of chronic diseases (such as hypertension and diabetes) has prompted Big Pharma, as well as consumer-packaged-goods companies, to buy their way into the supplement space. For food giants like Nestlé and Dannon, a push toward nutraceuticals was especially attractive because of the positive marketing spin to be gained from foods designed for health. And while a 25-percent margin on nutraceuticals might be less than what Big Pharma is used to getting from drug products, they still offer diversification without the investment that new drugs require. Nestlé bought PowerBar, Procter & Gamble acquired New Chapter, and Pfizer acquired Alacer Corp., just to name a few of the many high-profile acquisitions that came in to disrupt the natural supplement industry. Prior to Big Pharma's entry, natural supplements had been made by small companies specializing in niche nutritional products. There was little development effort, since natural molecules generally cannot be patented and their investment could never be recouped.

The tradeshow reflected this extreme fragmentation of the industry, with big players showcasing huge, brightly lighted tents, graced by identically dressed hostesses navigating their professionally staged décors, alongside simple tables manned by a single individual handing out leaflets.

A large, particularly eye-catching booth stole my attention. It looked like a Disney interpretation of a French winery, decorated in purple and earthy tones. Fake plastic grapes where hanging everywhere.

"Have you heard of resveratrol?"

A young woman in scanty purple dress was leaning over a makeshift table made of fake half barrels, "It is the reason why the French eat pastry, and cheese, and butter, and stay slim and healthy," she continued, without waiting for my answer.

"Well, I am French," I smiled, "and I can tell you that we do not get our resveratrol in the form of a supplement in France."

"Would you like to give it a try? It has all the antioxidant benefits of red wine, without the alcohol content." She handed me a little cup half-filled with purple liquid. "It is all-natural and delicious."

"You mean, kind of a grape juice?"

"Try it. It is all-natural and delicious." Obviously, her well-rehearsed selling points did not include an answer to my questions.

I took a sip, and could not refrain from wincing. "Yuck! This is pure, undiluted, syrup! Who can drink that? How can you pretend that this high-sugar concentrate is healthy?"

She quickly took the cup from my hands and looking far above my head said in a superior tone, "We like it sweet here."

I turned around. From the other side of the alley, a gentleman dressed as Uncle Sam, sporting a star-studded top hat and a red, white, and blue striped suit, was watching. He seemed to enjoy the scene. He was standing next to an older man who was manning the most basic booth—a table covered in black velvet with stacks of products on display.

"They just don't know how to make anything healthy," whispered Uncle Sam, with a vague hand gesture in direction of the fake winery, "They are allowed to sell their diabetes-enhancing piece of sh-t, excuse my French. They can even freely advertise their crap to kids—which should legally qualify as child abuse—while my friend Bob (gesture towards the older gentleman) has great supplements, really good for you, but he cannot even begin to tell you what they are for. And that is why it is most important for all of us to sign this petition to support the recognition of the freedom of speech for supplements as part of the First Amendment," he concluded, while already flashing a notepad in front of my eyes to collect signatures.

"Is this a joke?" I couldn't help asking, "I thought that America was founded on the principles of freedom and individual rights."

"In theory, yes, this is correct. The First Amendment to the U.S. Constitution reads in part: 'Congress shall make no law […] abridging the freedom of speech.' However, drug multinationals, whose main objective is profits, have bought out the politicians to rob us of our rights. And because dietary supplements are not permitted to diagnose, treat, cure, or prevent any disease or condition, dietary supplement companies cannot use even legitimate scientific information if the studies have been conducted on anyone with a disease or medical condition.

"Your school teacher told you about Christopher Columbus, right? Columbus told his crew to eat oranges to avoid scurvy. Well, nowadays, Christopher Columbus would possibly face jail time for such a statement! Every day, Americans are denied access to the very information they need to make informed lifestyle and health care decisions. And that is why it is so important to sign this petition and support freedom of speech and access to scientific information. Americans need to exercise independent judgment in caring for themselves."

"He's right," added the older gentleman, "I came to the tradeshow without any marketing material. Too dangerous."

I signed the petition page and continued walking.

But I kept thinking, *is this for real?*

In France, my father was forbidden to publish, and here legitimate companies were not allowed to use scientific publications!

If modern science was born out of the struggle between Galileo and the authorities for the right to express scientific ideas, not much progress has been made since the 16th century, either in France, the self-proclaimed champion of human rights, or in the United States, the first modern democracy!

I searched for Ken as I continued contemplating the apparent Dark Ages for the freedom of scientific expression. Finally, I found him mingling, laughing with a petite brunette on the far side of the room. As he saw me approaching, Ken straightened up.

"Hi there," he said casually, "Say hello to Juliette."

I pardoned the interruption and introduced myself as Ken's wife.

The petite brunette's brows arched slightly, but without missing a beat she extended her hand and introduced herself as one of the lead doctors associated with Cancer Treatment Centers of America® (CTCA®). She explained that the reason for her organization's attendance at the trade show was to create possible partnerships with companies who were interested in doing research.

"Excellent!" I responded. Immediately my antennae began to quiver. I explained that we had a unique compound that had already demonstrated its ability to offer valuable support to the production of white blood cells and platelets in previous animal studies, but that more research was needed to better ascertain its full potential. I was gambling with the idea that my mother and Bernard Fourche would be able to quickly come up with a way to manufacture the RNA fragments.

"Indeed, at CTCA, we have a lot of patients who receive chemotherapy, and some get thrombocytopenia (a condition that develops because of an abnormal loss of platelets in the blood) as a side effect of chemotherapy," she replied while reaching for a business card.

"When patients don't have enough platelets they tend to bleed a lot. So when they are losing too many platelets, we have to stop their rounds of chemotherapy. Then the cancer is not addressed and it keeps growing. Thrombocytopenia is a real issue. Anything that could help would be seriously considered."

"The RNA fragments help maintain a normal level of platelets." I stressed (Having heard Uncle Sam's speech, I insisted on "normal"), "You will not have to wait for thrombocytopenia to occur to see the benefits."

She seemed interested. We exchanged cards, and I stored hers preciously.

I somehow *knew* that it was important.

I had planned to meet with Dr. Schachter later at the hotel bar. His practice had been the recipient of most of the extracts received from Fourche. Although Dr. Schachter had many of his patients also taking several other products, he had been able to link marked improvements to the time when Beljanski's extracts had been added to their regimen.

Dr. Schachter's offer to present my father's work at a medical conference was a major breakthrough in terms of international recognition. I was very excited, and couldn't dream of a better spokesperson for Beljanski's work.

It was still early for our appointment, but I was feeling tired and decided to go wait at the bar. In the middle of a sea of gaming tables and slot machines, a floating, ornate, red and gold Hollywood version of a pharaonic barge (nothing like the tiny craft on the Rio Negro), seemed like an inviting setting to unwind. I headed towards it.

"Hello from Julius Caesar!"

A red-haired, blue-eyed Julius Caesar in a tunic, lending his arm to a chunky Cleopatra with a gaudy tiara, was waving at clients. I couldn't help but smile.

As the improbable couple walked away, I remember thinking: *If I end up losing everything in this adventure, I can always apply for this kind of job.*

Finally Dr. Schachter arrived. We warmly greeted each other, and he immediately got down to business. He confirmed that he had had very good results applying the botanical extracts to several of his patients. He had started with one suffering from advanced pancreatic cancer, who, against all odds, began to get better after *Pao pereira* and *Rauwolfia vomitoria* were added to his regimen. From there, Dr. Schachter added the extracts to the regimen of several other advanced cancer patients suffering from different kinds of cancer and noted their improvements as well.

"I think that I have enough solid material for a conference and to write a piece in the Health Letter of FAIM (Foundation for Alternative Integrative Medicine)," he concluded.

I was elated.

At that moment, my telephone rang, and Gérard's name popped up on the screen. I knew it was very early in the morning in France, so it had to be important.

Ignoring Ken's look of disapproval, I asked to be excused so I could take the call. It was difficult to find a quiet spot in the middle of a casino filled with people and music, so I made my way to the ladies' room and pressed myself into an empty corner.

"Yes, Gérard?" I strained to hear his voice above the incessant chatter of the women refreshing themselves.

"Bernard Fourche is dead!" Gérard's voice was trembling.

"What?"

My first thought was that because of the level of surrounding noise, I had not heard correctly.

"Car accident...That's all I know for now."

I tried to take a deep breath, but my chest was constricting and the intense panic that immediately followed my comprehension of his words was overwhelming. I had met Fourche only once. But because of his help in providing me with the first batches of extracts, the trust that he had put in me, his willingness to carry on with the production of the products, it felt like I had lost a family member.

The enormity of what I had embarked upon struck me. Here we were, a family of souls all involved in serving this project that was bigger than any of us: salvaging what could possibly be a natural solution to cancer! Everything done so far relied on the premise that Bernard Fourche would be involved in producing the extracts, or at least overseeing their manufacturing. Without a consistent production, this entire enterprise was doomed.

Don't show your anxiety! whispered a small internal voice.

Painfully, I filled my lungs with air and then let it out, slowly, slowly. And then another.

I was starting to feel light-headed. I needed to sit down. Despite a dry mouth, dry throat, and pounding heart, I managed to get back to our table, order a Caracalla drink, and wear a smile the rest of the evening.

Inside I felt like a zombie.

––––––––––––––

I called Gérard back as soon as I could.

"Any other news?" I asked, this time my voice trembling. He had none. I abruptly changed the topic.

"Do you have an idea of how much the lab might weigh?" I asked, remembering Ken's earlier derogatory remark about the value of the laboratory equipment.

"Huh? You mean the centrifuge, the computers, and microscopes? No, I have no idea. Why? Nobody ever weighs those kinds of things!"

"Do you think you could convince the receiver that it is all old, outdated stuff, worth the value of the metal scraps, and that he will be lucky if he finds a buyer for a few thousand dollars?"

"I don't know," said Gérard. "And it is not true! Just last year we spent a small fortune on the freeze dryer alone! And the centrifuge is huge. I am sure that it is also quite expensive."

"Well, if you had to guess a total weight, what would be your best guess?"

"I have no idea..." he insisted, "Maybe 500 kg? ... or 800?"

"Okay," I said, "Listen, I can scrape together a budget of $3,000. Tell the receiver that you have an American client willing to pay cash $3/kg for a total of 1,000kgs, and let's see what happens."

"I've never heard of anything like that, but I can try," offered Gérard. He paused, "And then, if you get it, what are you going to do with it?"

"I'll get back to you," I told him. "Let's first see what the receiver has to say about the offer."

I knew that often (at least in France) cash is king with court-appointed receivers. They are much more eager to move quickly to their next file than to secure real value for the assets they are in charge of liquidating.

Two weeks later, my all-cash offer had indeed been accepted by the receiver. No questions asked. Nobody else had made a higher offer. I had to admit that Ken had been right regarding the low value of second-hand laboratory equipment.

A month later, I had secured a place in New Jersey suitable for a small laboratory. Two months after that, a huge container filled with laboratory equipment and state-of-the-art machinery was delivered all the way from Burgundy, France. Several people, including a handful of scientists close to my parents, flew in to help. I have to give very special thanks here to Mr. Guilbert, who was initially scheduled to work for Bernard Fourche, and came to New Jersey to help set up the lab.

"Oh my gosh!" he exclaimed as he plugged in the HPLC system. Short for High Performance Liquid Chromatography, the device is a sophisticated, expensive instrument used to separate, identify, and quantify each of the compounds that are present in a sample. HPLC testing is a necessity to meet the increasingly stringent quality standards and the demands of regulatory authorities around the world.

"What is it?" I asked.

"All the quality control values, all the material specifications—it is all there, in the HPLC's computer. They gave it to you loaded with all the chromatograms of all the testing records! You now have all the analytical methods you need to characterize the safety, identity, purity, composition, authenticity, and origin of all of your father's products."

He then proceeded to open a small black box filled with little vials.

"And here!" he pronounced, " All the reference materials you need! Madame, I am telling you, you hit the jackpot! This data is far more valuable than the computer itself!"

My heart skipped a beat.

"I collected some little flecks of bark from the Botanical Garden of Rio de Janeiro," I said breathlessly, "Can we test how rich they are in flavopereirine? That's the active molecule to which my father had attributed the activity of his *Pao pereira* extract.

"Sure!" exclaimed Mr. Guilbert with a wide grin. "You can test the raw materials, the finished products, and everything in between."

Thanks to this unexpected windfall of data, I could now approach reputable manufacturing companies and check if their extracts were able to match my father's in purity and strength. Within a matter of months, I would be able to entrust a good American company with taking over the production of the products that my father had perfected in France. I also envisioned The Beljanski Foundation establishing itself as an independent reference for the quality of those products, should they become popular one day, with several manufacturers competing for the same market.*

While new life was being injected into Beljanski's discoveries in the U.S., closure was finally obtained in France. As noted previously, in 2002 a unanimous decision was reached by the European Court of Human Rights in the case *Beljanski*

---

*   See Appendix 2: *Pao pereira* content comparison chart (Flavopereirine) *vs. France.*[5] We won, but it was a bittersweet victory after a protracted four-year battle. Surprisingly, however, it had not been a hard one to win from a legal point of view. From the beginning it had been clear that the French General Attorney had no case. That did not prevent him from delaying as long as the process would allow, making the trial as emotionally difficult and expensive for my family as he could. The arguments presented on behalf of the French government had been consistently and shockingly poor. I was relieved we had won, but as a French lawyer, I was profoundly ashamed by France's public display of such intense mediocrity.

Shortly thereafter Dr. Schachter published his piece in FAIM. It was a very thorough review of my father's work, entitled "Mirko Beljanski's Innovative Approach to Cancer, Chronic Viral Diseases and Auto Immune Conditions."[6]

The first American paper about my father's work! I felt like I could literally touch international recognition! I was so grateful to Dr. Schachter, and to America, and was beyond ecstatic! I felt the urge to share the news with everybody I knew, including the doorman, the dry cleaner, the dentist, the banker. Nobody was spared from receiving a copy of Dr. Schachter's article, along with my outpouring of enthusiasm.

Little did I know that my banker was a patient of Dr. Aaron Katz, head of the Department of Holistic Urology at Columbia University at the time. As a result, a few weeks later, I received *the* call.

"Hello?"

"Hi, this is Dr. Katz at Columbia," responded the deep, sexy voice, "A paper about your father—I guess, is that right?—has come to my attention. There might be some interest for us here. I am eager to learn more about it. Would you like to come to Columbia to provide me with more details?"

I was swept away, but also apprehensive. I knew that without a scientific background I sorely lacked credibility. My enthusiasm for my father's work could quickly turn into a liability if I were perceived as nothing more than a sweet "Daddy's little girl" with an unresolved Oedipus complex. If people were going to reject me as the messenger, then the message would not be received, and this fantastic opportunity to address cancer would be lost for all humankind.

I need to bring credibility to the process, I thought. *But how?*

The next Sunday morning, I was trying to relax while reading the *New York Times*. It was an impossible task, since I couldn't seem to get my mission out of my mind. As I aimlessly turned the pages of the newspaper, my attention was suddenly captured by the page in front of me.

"That's it!" I exclaimed, "I am going to place an ad in the classifieds for a scientist."

And that's just what I did.

Two weeks later, I was poring over the resumes that I had received, when one really caught my eye. It belonged to Dr. John Hall, who had a PhD in molecular biology, just like my father. He had gotten his degree from New York University in the very same department where my father had spent his two-year fellowship with Nobel prize recipient Severo Ochoa before returning to the Pasteur Institute in Paris, France.

I called him to set up an interview.

When I first opened the door, his full white beard and hearty demeanor made me think of Santa Claus. *Santa Claus with a PhD?* That seemed good to me. But I knew that I still had to persuade him that The Beljanski Foundation would serve his professional ambition.

In an effort to win him over, I tried to summarize my father's work. I tentatively expressed something along the lines of what Dr. Devra Davis would brilliantly write later in the foreword of my father's book, which would later be reprinted in the U.S.:

> "The limits of conventional treatments for cancer and other chronic diseases are evident in the failure to achieve significant advances in the survival of many forms of cancer [...] In his pioneering work in France and the United States more than half a century ago, Mirko Beljanski laid the foundation for understanding what today is termed epigenetic. Beljanski studied how external factors can interact directly with DNA, causing structural changes and the initiation of cancers without having any impact on the genetic code itself [...] Those on the cutting edge of clinical work today are indebted to Beljanski for forging new approaches to evaluating the role of various interventions and supplements [...] In recent years, epigenetics has become one of the most dynamic and vibrant areas in biomedical sciences."[7]

I could feel that Dr. Hall was still quite skeptical. I placed before him Dr. Schachter's recent paper,[6] as well as the stack of 133 Beljanski publications (including the one posthumously published by *Genetics and Molecular Biology*,[8] evidencing how the same natural compound may be effective to fight many different forms of cancer.

Dr. Hall's eyes widened as he flipped through the materials.

Finally, I thought with some relief.

"This is not mainstream," he said, "However it's definitively worth looking into. It's funny, I was recently looking into the work of another scientist, D.C. Malins.[9] His team at the Pacific Northwest Research Foundation has recently confirmed this work while using contemporary technology. Malins called the carcinogen-induced structural changes in DNA 'disorders,' but this is basically the same thing as 'destabilization of the primary structure of the DNA' termed by Beljanski."

He was quiet for some time, which felt like an eternity to me, as he looked through the documents.

"I will need some time to look into this," he finally stated.

"I will need your answer very fast," I replied, "We have a meeting at Columbia University next week."

CHAPTER SEVEN
ALL OVER AGAIN

"Most allopathic doctors think practitioners of alternative medicine are all quacks. They're not. Often they're sharp people who think differently about disease."

DR. MEHMET OZ

M any times, it's easiest to just give up. But consider the spider that toils on relentlessly... through the night and through the rain until the web is built. And if something comes along and destroys his or her beautiful creation, the diligent spider begins to build again....

Columbia University is a private Ivy League research university, located on a park-like campus in the Morningside Heights neighborhood of upper Manhattan.

The campus was bustling with student activity the day we visited, and I couldn't stop watching everything around me. It was so different from the Sorbonne in Paris where I studied! The Sorbonne is in the heart of the city and has no campus. The building of the Sorbonne itself, built in the thirteenth century, exudes history and restraint.

There I was at Columbia, the famous university, with a precious copy of my father's publications safely tucked away in my attaché case.

At first, I was surprised by how young Dr. Katz looked. Another refreshing departure from the usual fatherly French teaching figures. Flashing a perfect smile, he explained how he came to oversee the Holistic Urology Department. As a Professor of Urology at Columbia University Hospital College of Physicians and Surgeons, Dr. Katz had been trained as a conventional medical doctor. He also had the opportunity to work at an integrative medicine center in New York City (the Atkins Center). There he saw that many of the patients using vitamins, herbs, and nutrition felt much better at a time when he would have thought they should have had surgery. He soon became an advocate for integrative medicine.

"Doctors get so focused on looking at their one area of expertise and that is where holistic medicine is different," he explained. "We look at the whole body, and treat patients individually. A holistic approach has very little risk and offers great benefits for the majority of patients. It's not just about monitoring your blood test, it's also about incorporating some terrific evidence-based approaches and enlarging your treatment options. It offers the best of both worlds—the best of conventional medicine and the best of alternative medicine. I am one of the few urologists involved in clinical and laboratory studies of natural formulas, so I see firsthand the very best and the truly worst on both sides."

Dr. Katz pointed out that prostate cancer is among the most prevalent cancers in men. It is estimated that one out of six men will get prostate cancer, and one out of thirty-four will die from the disease.[1] These numbers indicate that many men will go on living with prostate cancer and die of other causes. The fact that most prostate cancers advance slowly makes the disease an excellent model for holistic medicine where conventional treatments are combined with alternative therapies, focusing on supporting prostate health and preventing the development of a more aggressive disease.

I found Dr. Katz to be very open-minded and eager to hear about any new plant extract that could contribute to the well-being of his patients. Dr. Hall and myself explained that Beljanski had found that certain natural molecules could specifically recognize and bind to the destabilized DNA that has been exposed to carcinogens, thereby inhibiting the replication of abnormal DNA. Although he never published anything specifically on prostate cancer, prostate cancer was included in the sixteen different kinds of cancer cell lines that his research showed *Pao pereira* was working on.[2]

I told Dr. Katz about President Mitterrand, and how a mixture of *Pao pereira* and *Rauwolfia vomitoria* extracts had helped him contain his advanced prostate cancer for several years.

Throughout our conversation, Dr. Katz gave us his undivided attention, nodding at intervals to let us know he understood exactly what we were saying. I was extremely grateful and honored to have his audience because I knew he was a very busy man with many important matters to attend to. I was pleased to hear him say how impressed he was with the quality of the scientific journals in which my father had published.

Then he stood up and began to pace the floor, appearing deep in thought.

"Very interesting," he muttered after a while, as he continued his walk across the tiled floor of the sparsely decorated office. After a few more moments, he returned to his seat across from me.

"Very interesting," he repeated, "*But...*"

He leaned back in his chair, and I leaned forward to hear what this "*but*"—obviously, an obstacle—was all about.

"But," he continued, "Columbia University is an outstanding research university with tremendous clout. It's not that I don't believe you, but I cannot give something to my patients that has not first been thoroughly tested by this university. I appreciate that the toxicology studies have been done, but I will nonetheless need to test the product myself first in vitro, and then if everything goes well, in vivo with mice, before we can move forward with my patients."

I really don't know how to explain what I was feeling.

Disappointment?

Anxiety?

Dismay?

Outrage?

Confusion?

All the above?

I squealed, "So you mean that despite all the French publications, the French mice, all the French doctors who have been recommending the products for years, all the patients who have done well taking the products, including the French president, we have to return to square one with the American in vitro cell essays? And then follow up with American mice?! All over again? This is going to take forever..."

"No, not forever. If all goes well, it will only be a matter of months, and we can begin as soon as you are ready."

The flashy smile was back. Dr. Katz had laid out his concerns and conditions, and *this* was the course that had to be taken before any consideration could be given to administering the products to his patients.

Dr. Hall turned to me, "Since your father did not specifically publish any research on prostate cancer, this is a wonderful opportunity to confirm that those extracts are effectively working on that specific cancer, and get all the data. You can't dream of a better form of recognition than a publication from Columbia's Department of Urology."

For a few seconds, I struggled to put aside emotions and think positively: *At least Dr. Katz was willing to give it a try.* And recognition was now in the cards. It was only a matter of time.

"So," Dr. Katz's deep voice interrupted my inward struggle, "Which product do you think will work best? *Pao pereira* or *Rauwolfia vomitoria?*"

I chuckled despite my frustration. He was ready to move forward and apparently wasn't giving me any option besides moving forward with him.

It's settled then.

I let Dr. Katz know that both products worked equally well against cancer cells, although they had slightly different properties: *Rauwolfia* was a favorite for hormonal-dependent tissues (like prostate), while *Pao pereira* was very versatile and seemed to have anti-inflammatory and antiviral benefits as well. We concluded that we would investigate the extracts separately to collect quality data from each one.

And so, the research into the anticancer effects of the *Pao pereira* and *Rauwolfia vomitoria* extracts at Columbia University Medical Center began under the direction of Dr. Aaron Katz and his colleague Dr. Debra Bemis.

The initial batches provided by Fourche were by now long gone, and only American-made extracts were available for the Columbia studies. I felt a little pinch of anxiety. *Will the American-made extract deliver as well as my father's? Will Dr. Katz and his team be able to reproduce and confirm the results from the Pasteur Institute?*

The results turned out to be conclusive, as I had hoped. Using rigorous tests in vitro (cell-based studies), they showed that the extracts inhibit the growth of human prostate cancer cells (LNCaP) by inducing either apoptosis (cell death) or cell cycle arrest (also leading to cell death). These were both very attractive mechanisms of action for anticancer agents, handsomely completing what my father had been able to assess in France in his own laboratory.

Pleased with the in vitro results, Columbia went on to conduct in vivo studies and—as expected—American mice responded the same as French mice. In the presence of both extracts, their tumors were significantly shrinking. In some cases, tumor growth was suppressed by up to 80 percent!

Columbia University published its results, both on *Pao pereira*[3] and on *Rauwolfia vomitoria*,[4] demonstrating the efficacy, as well as the safety, of both plant extracts and confirming the claims my father originally made.

It also meant that the extracts, now made in America according to Beljanski's specific methodology, were just as good as those originally made in France during my father's time. My father was gone, but his know-how had survived. The destructive wrath of the French government was no match for the truth! Just like a fragile little cutting, freshly planted, Beljanski's legacy was now ready to take root and flourish in a new land.

And isn't America dubbed the land of second chances?

Columbia's team went on to study the synergy of action of both extracts with the chemotherapy drug docetaxel, which is the drug most often used in America to treat prostate cancer. When my father was at the Pasteur Institute he had tested the synergy of action of his extracts with several of the chemotherapy drugs commonly used at the time (including "5FU" and "Endoxan"), but those drugs had not included docetaxel. Each chemotherapy drug is a different molecule and a nice synergy with one does not necessarily ensure the same synergy with another. So it was quite a relief to see that it was working with docetaxel as well.

I felt the need to share my joy with the Heart of Palm Lady in Brazil.

When we spoke, she had great news to share as well.

Even though the *Pao pereira* tree exhibits a great regenerative capacity in the wild, she had decided to ensure 100 percent sustainability of her operation and grow her own trees on a piece of land far more accessible than the remote village we had visited. With a germination rate of over 50 percent usually achieved within a month or so, she had managed to create a nursery of about *two hundred* saplings. She had only been waiting for their first leaves to take pictures and break the news!

I had to fly back to Brazil. I couldn't wait to see all these little "*Pao* babies" myself.

My visit to the nursery was filled with emotion. Any manifestation of the vitality of life appeals to our survival instinct and brings us joy, but a nursery of cancer-fighting trees... that was the picture of hope for the future of humankind! The epitome of goodness!

The bright, tiny, green leaves were perfectly identical in shape to the darker green leaves I had observed on the grown trees at the Rio de Janeiro botanical garden. They were all just perfect little babies!

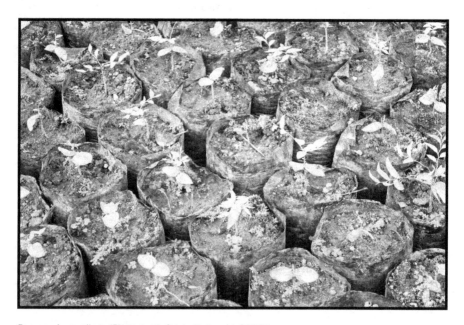

Pao pereira saplings (Photograph Sylvie Beljanski, 2003.)

The Columbia publications arrived on the heels of the presentation that Dr. Schachter gave about Beljanski's work to fellow American physicians at the American College for Advancement in Medicine (ACAM) in Washington D.C. For years Dr. Schachter had been extremely active in the field of alternative and complementary medicine, and he is highly regarded by his peers. He served as vice-president of the Academy of Orthomolecular Psychiatry (AOP), president of the American College for Advancement of Medicine (ACAM), and president of the Foundation for the Advancement of Innovative Medicine.

Addressing a packed audience, he explained, "The magnitude of Beljanski's findings struck me as being significant. They were so well researched. I have always felt the current paradigm only barely scratched the surface of our understanding of the true causes and most successful approaches to cancer. As I was impressed with Dr. Beljanski's work, I decided to share this information, since his work is virtually unknown in the United States."

Dr. Schachter continued by offering a masterful summary of my father's fifty years of research. Then he concluded: "To summarize, the research work of Mirko Beljanski led to the development of four nutritional supplements that are potentially beneficial to cancer patients, either alone or in combination with conventional treatments. Two of them (extracts of *Pao pereira* and *Rauwolfia vomitoria*) have selective anticancer activity, meaning that they selectively damage cancer cells, but not normal cells. One of them (RNA fragments from nonpathogenic E. coli) is useful for stimulating all types of normal white blood cells and platelets, and is particularly beneficial for patients undergoing radiation and/or chemotherapy. Finally, the last one, a special extract from *Ginkgo Biloba,* has been used as a nutritional supplement to help prevent abnormal scar tissue formation from radiation or surgery."[5]

Dr. Schachter's conference was very well received by health professionals. Shortly after, I was approached almost simultaneously by Dr. Stephen Coles, a Visiting Scholar at UCLA and director of the Supercentenarian Research Foundation, and by Dr. Morton Walker, the famed recipient of twenty-three medical journalism awards, author of two thousand clinical articles and ninety-two published books. They both indicated their interest in writing about my father and his research, but their projects were quite different. Dr. Coles was leaning towards an historical depiction of my father's life, stressing how his dramatic and compelling story illustrated the way bureaucratic agendas place politics above scientific truth, at the expense of the knowledge necessary to extend human life.[6] On the other hand, Dr. Walker wanted to educate the public about "a scientifically proven way to handle cancer that didn't kill the patient" as he later explained in his preface to the book *Cancer's Cause, Cancer's Cure*:

> "Nearly ten years ago, I retired from my active participation in medical journalism. But when cancer took my wife, my mother, my sister, and my fiancée who had pledged to spend her last years with me, I knew I had to step up and not only uncover which alternatives really worked, but also let the world know about it."[7]

The more the merrier, I thought. I pledged to help them both by providing open access to all the documents that my mother and I had been systematically retrieving and collecting since my father's passing. My mother especially extended herself relentlessly for several months, answering any questions they both had.

Both books intended to mention how the Beljanski legacy was carried to America through the pursuit of high-profile additional research, and how the Columbia University publications validated my father's previous results.

The pressure was on to get even more results.

Dr. Katz and I decided to meet in midtown near the Columbia University Medical Center after one of his consultations. I still remember the perfect early summer day and that I was wearing a flowery dress and open-toed shoes. I decided to take a stroll and was walking towards the restaurant when I felt my phone buzz in my shoulder bag. My Heart of Palm Lady was calling from Brazil. She was in tears and I stopped in the middle of the street.

"The Federal Police has come to my place… They have seized everything that I've collected for the past five months. They claim that the authorizations I received from the Ministry of Agriculture are not recognized by the Ministry of Forests, that I am selling the Amazon to some big American company, and they want me to pay a big fine or to go to jail for it. But I have not done anything illegal! I swear on my daughter's life! I have all the papers! They are the criminals. What they want is to grab my land. They put us out of business. It's all about mahogany. They are building this big dam, and now all the big mahogany loggers are paying off the police to come and push us out—"

"What about the *Pao* nursery?"

"You don't understand, it's all gone!" she cried. "When they want to take over your land, they declare that you have no right to grow your crop and they destroy it. Once you are ruined, they assess a huge fine! The only way to pay for these huge fines is to give them the land or go to jail!"

In that moment, it felt like a giant octopus was squeezing my heart and stomach. At the same time, there was a strange feeling of disbelief and *déjà vu. Would governmental greed prevent the development of what I now believed was the most serious natural treatment for cancer?*

Forest law cannot be effectively enforced in the absence of good governance. Where corruption is widespread, government funds allocated to the conservation of natural resources are often embezzled. Several large hydroelectric projects, funded without thorough review of their environmental impact by international development organizations like the World Bank, have led to massive rainforest loss. Besides clearing away large tracts of rainforest and killing off local wildlife, they have destroyed aquatic habitats and affected fish populations, displacing indigenous peoples, and adding carbon to the atmosphere as the submerged wood rots.

Brazil's former 'mahogany belt,' a region rich in rare and wonderful wood species, was an area of enormous ecological diversity that stretched over some eighty million hectares. It has now become the Amazon's "deforestation belt." The Belo Monte dam, sold to the public as a source of "clean energy," is slated to be the third largest hydroelectric project in the world. It is poised to divert 80 percent of the Xingu River's flow through artificial canals, flooding an area larger than Chicago while drying out other areas that are home to hundreds of indigenous and riverine families. The plan is to use the power to run bauxite, iron, gold, and copper smelters.

Construction of this massive $18 billion project has caused the forced relocation of up to forty thousand people. Illegality and corruption in forest management run high through bribes, as harvesters with money and connections buy their access to forest activities, and, consequently, deny access to others with fewer economic and social resources.

Greenpeace once documented how a huge log-yard on the Kayapó land, on the left bank of the Xingu River, has devastated the area with trucks, cars, bulldozers and a large logging road leading into the forest. "The forestry elite dominates communal institutions through intimidation, manipulating elections, dodging oversight, and discouraging participation in community assemblies," reads a report by the World Wildlife Foundation.[8]

Who benefits?

At one point, it was reported that half to two-thirds of U.K.'s imported timber was coming from such illegal sources[9], some of it under the umbrella of the French multinational Saint Gobain.[10]

In addition to the large-scale grand corruption undermining the substantial stringency of forest laws, there are many "small fish," such as illegal loggers who also contribute to deforestation, mostly by ranching. Illegal cattle pastures have been the active focus of public prosecutors and federal police, but the system itself, by all accounts, is weakened by corruption and legal loopholes.

Even though it all seemed unreal, I believed my Heart of Palm Lady's story. Her respect for the local tribes had been obvious to me, as well as her genuine desire to provide them with essential income through fair trade. Harvesting of the *Pao pereira* bark can be done without cutting down the trees, and the bark regenerates quickly. Additionally, the carbon footprints of a simple boat or a donkey are minimal. Finally, her raising the nursery of little *Pao* saplings had revealed the full extent of her commitment to sustainability.

Deep down, I knew that none of this would be relevant to her case, and that she had little- to-no chance of winning her legal battle. I asked her to let me know how I could help, but she was too emotional to provide me with any concrete answers. Even if she managed to pay the fine, it would only be a matter of time before they assess another one, under whatever pretense they could come up with.

I was crushed by the news, but I had little time to dwell on my feelings. I was still headed to my lunch appointment with Dr. Katz at Columbia University to discuss a research program. And now I had no secured pipeline of product.

What should I say? Should I cancel the research program altogether?

My little internal voice came back and told me to keep my chin up and trust that the universe would provide.

At the restaurant, Dr. Katz greeted me with his trademark flashy grin. Despite my anxiety I smiled back. He reiterated his enthusiasm for the safety and efficacy displayed by both extracts in the initial studies.[3,4] Having shown that tumor growth was suppressed by up to 80 percent in mice grafted with prostate tumor cells and with no signs of toxicity, Dr. Katz was now ready to run a clinical trial on men with an elevated PSA reading. He would give them a special combination of both *Pao pereira* and *Rauwolfia Vomitoria*. Indeed, whenever two anticancer agents work by different mechanisms of action, it makes sense to use them together. This approach takes advantage of the potential for a synergistic effect, especially considering that there are not many treatment options currently offered to men with elevated PSA. Typically, such patients are put on regular observation of their condition, waiting for the time when conventional treatment (radiation, chemotherapy and surgery) becomes necessary.

A clinical trial on men will require an awful lot of capsules, I thought. I felt chills down my back. I could barely touch my plate, but I resisted sharing my inventory problems with Dr. Katz.

Instead I said "This sounds great, but my concern is that it will take a very long time to put a clinical trial in place. I assume that you will have to run the project by Columbia University's Institution Review Board. They may take forever to approve this project."

"I hear you," he answered, "There is always the risk of some major administrative delays. Alternatively, we could conduct another in vitro essay regarding the effectiveness of both extracts on those advanced prostate cancer cells (CRPC PC3 cells) that do not answer any longer to hormonal treatments."

For men suffering from prostate cancer metastasis, the standard treatment is castration therapy. This emasculating treatment comes with many devastating side effects, and it's common knowledge that it can't cure the cancer. The point of knocking the testosterone level down towards zero is to temporarily halt the progression of prostate cancer. But testosterone does not cause cancer, it only fuels it. Castration is effective at slowing down the progression of the cancer, but only until it stops working. Then the cancer wins. And when hormonal therapy fails, men are out of options. There is no curative treatment for those patients at that stage.

Dr. Katz continued, "Inflammation is intimately linked to the activation of NFκB, increasing the expression of anti-apoptotic, proliferative, and metastatic proteins in prostate cancer.[11] You told me that your father had observed that *Pao pereira* had some anti-inflammatory effect, in addition to its anticancer effect?"

"That's right," I answered, "My father credited that activity to the improvement reported by many people suffering from brain cancer."[12]

"Brain? The same product used for prostate?"

"Absolutely. My father's last paper showed that the extract's activity is not organ- or gender-specific."[2]

"Well, it would be great to know if *Pao pereira* exhibits anticancer properties against those cancer cells which have become castration-resistant. If we could be the first to report that the *Pao pereira* extract has anticancer effects against highly malignant metastatic CRPC PC3 cells, that would be a major breakthrough."

The prospect of a major breakthrough, coupled with the need to provide Dr. Katz only with the limited amount of extract that an in vitro essay requires, made this look like the perfect project: We agreed to go ahead with the research program on advanced prostate cancer cells.

An invention must be new to be patentable. That is why pharmaceutical and biotech companies invest so heavily in creating new-to-nature molecules they can successfully patent, thereby securing a monopoly on the product and its profits. Natural substances are not new and therefore are not patentable. The same herbs are often available through different companies, all competing for a piece of market share. From one company to another, the bottles may look somewhat similar, but there can be a wide difference of potency between the extracts, and the labels rarely offer clear readings. As Dr. Katz puts it, "A lot of companies are trying to make a quick dollar on this hugely popular herbal healer, but only a few are paying attention to producing a quality product that really works."[13]

I was aware that several companies were selling varieties of *Pao pereira* extracts, both in the U.S. and Europe. I figured that with our Brazilian supplier gone, The Beljanski Foundation ought to collect samples from these companies and see if any could provide an alternative source of material for research.

In the process, I was shocked to discover that several of those companies were using my father's name and quoting his research to promote their products, sometimes with outlandish claims.

I had The Beljanski Foundation make anonymous orders of several *Pao pereira* extracts from various companies selling across Europe (Luxembourg, Belgium, Spain, etc.), the U.S., and Canada. All the products were stored, analyzed under identical conditions, and evaluated by a certified laboratory specializing in quality control. For each sample, we wanted to measure the amount of flavopereirine, the active compound in *Pao pereira*.

Compared to the data that had come with my father's salvaged laboratory equipment, it was clear that the concentration of flavopereirine used in the products sold by nearly all these companies was far inferior to the one used by Mirko Beljanski when conducting his research. There was one exception: Natural Source International, the New York-based company that had provided all the samples used by Columbia University for its research.

There was no other viable alternative. Given how difficult it had been to source the Heart of Palm Lady as a reliable provider in the first place, a shortage of product was most likely to come.

———————

The yearly CIRIS picnic has been a tradition since 1991. On the first weekend of each September, several hundred people come from all over the country to gather in an open-air, beautiful yet informal garden of a 17th century Carmel convent named Notre-Dame-de-Recouvrance, in the French city of Saintes. This timeless and stunning backdrop is the setting for a great day of friendship and emotional support. Sharing is a positive, reinforcing, feel-good gesture for those who have been able to overcome their diagnoses, while those newly diagnosed are eager to receive every bit of information they can from those who have "made it."

This truly exceptional gathering rose to international fame in 2008 when a group photo of the participants graced the cover of the American magazine, *The Doctor's Prescription for Healthy Living*.

With Dr. Walker wishing to conduct his own inquiry and base his book on testimonials that he would collect himself directly from people who had suffered different kinds of cancers and credited my father's extracts for their survival, I invited him to come to the upcoming CIRIS picnic.

When the rumor spread that an American journalist was coming all the way from New York to write about them, dozens of CIRIS members expressed their eagerness to share with the world their journey through disease and recovery. There was no way that all the interviews could take place in a single day. Gérard and his wife Pierrette went beyond the call of duty to welcome Dr. Walker into their own home. They also hosted a long parade of people for three full days, with Gérard enforcing a strict twenty-minute interview rule, while generous Pierrette fed everybody delicious homemade organic food.

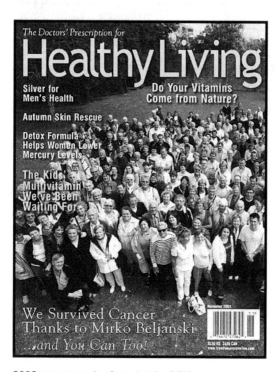

2008 cover magazine featuring the CIRIS picnic.

I was especially happy to reunite with Jean-Paul Le Perlier, whose skin color had evolved from its lemony hue to a healthier pinkish tone. He was obviously beating the odds, and his colon cancer diagnosis was now officially no longer terminal.

As all these people went on record to express their gratitude to my father, their candid testimonials often reflected in passing glimpses how we, as humans, cope with adversity.

"My prostate cancer is stabilized, even my knee arthritis is better... I decided to drive down and introduce my new fiancée to you all," said an eighty-three-year-old.

"My doctor didn't want me to take anything besides the chemotherapy, so I decided to do my own thing on the side without telling him. He is surprised by how well I'm doing, but as of today he still has no clue how I did it," said a breast cancer survivor who would not look us in the eyes while calmly explaining how she had defied medical authority.

"I said NO. Screw the hospital, screw the surgery, screw the cancer. And look at me. Here I am!" roared a very energetic brain cancer survivor.*

All of the testimonials were profoundly moving. I felt both proud and humbled that I had been given a chance to play a small part in their recovery.

But then again, how to tell them that after having succeeded almost miraculously in defying the shattering fury of the French government, their survival was now at risk because of a greedy and corrupted Brazilian government? How could I ever explain that a government had destroyed saplings in the name of environmental protection? I just couldn't bring myself to deliver the terrible news.

Instead I told them, "Next year I'll come back with a camera, and we'll make a documentary. I already have the footage of my father's last interview, filmed in my parent's dining room, and we could put that together and tell the great story of CIRIS."**

They loved the idea, and I wished with every fiber of my heart that I knew there would be a next year.

---

* Numerous testimonials are available at www.beljanski.org

** Movie "The Beljanski Legacy" available on the Beljanski Foundation's YouTube channel: https://www.youtube.com/watch?v=5dSz0bmwcj0

CHAPTER EIGHT
AND THE SCIENCE GOES ON

"Seems you can't outsmart Mother Nature."

DR. MARK HYMAN

G rowth and development go hand and hand. As a child grows, he or she takes on new challenges. That's development. The child can never run if he has not mastered the art of walking. Likewise, the caterpillar will not become a butterfly if he does not go through the process of transformation.

No wonder Chicago is called The Windy City, I thought, winding my fashionable-but-too-thin, wool scarf tightly around my neck while braving the frigid breezes blowing off Lake Michigan.

I was there to meet with doctors at the Illinois-based Cancer Treatment Centers of America (CTCA), a massive facility, part of a national network of five hospitals that serves about seventy-four hundred cancer-fighting patients per year. My visit could not have come at a better time. Indeed, after many administrative delays, Professor Shmuel Shoshan had finally published a study[1] on the risk of toxicity associated with the use of products like Neupogen and Neulasta, (commercial names for similar molecules: the granulocyte colony-stimulating factor, or G-CSF). These are widely recognized as the gold standard for fighting the depletion of white blood cells as a side effect of chemotherapy. His findings suggested that the administration of such products to healthy patients may be safe ... for five days!

Five days didn't sound like much.

Beyond those five days, Pr. Shoshan and his team found that DNA destabilization was significantly increased, and that this destabilization lasted for up to two months! Considering that DNA destabilization had been linked by both Beljanski and Malins to cancer formation, this was a subtle way of saying that these widely prescribed products might induce cancer when used beyond five days.

So much for the gold standard!

The study also marked the first time that the Oncotest (developed by Beljanski to measure levels of DNA destabilization,)[2] was officially reproduced and used in a hospital setting to measure the potential carcinogenicity of a product.

The scientific community didn't pick up on the Oncotest, but Shoshan's results on G-CSF drew a lot of interest. The issue of G-CSF's potentially detrimental long-term effects quickly became a major focus of international discussion and research.[3,4,5,6,7]

In addition to being highly toxic, G-CSF-based products are also extremely expensive. In 2017, one 6 mg Neulasta injection cost between $5,000 and $7,000, and one 300-microgram Neupogen injection cost between $300 and $350.[8] Neulasta is typically injected twenty-four hours after each cycle of high-dose chemotherapy, while Neupogen is typically injected daily until white blood cell counts come back to normal levels.

Finally, in addition to being toxic and expensive, the drugs work on white blood cells (treatment-induced anemia and neutropenia), but are not effective in preventing the loss of blood platelets* induced by chemotherapy. Radiotherapy and chemotherapy attack not only cancer cells but also the bone marrow where blood cells are manufactured, depleting the stem cells involved in both white blood cells and platelet proliferation. Thrombocytopenia, defined as platelet counts below 80,000 platelets/ml of blood, occurs when platelets are depleted from the bloodstream faster than they can be replaced. To fight the depletion of white blood cells, drugs like Neupogen or Neulasta are prescribed, but they don't

---

* Platelets are cell particles that are released into the bloodstream by the bone marrow, and are necessary to control bleeding and promote clotting. The normal blood platelet count ranges from 150,000 to 450,000 for every cubic millimeter of blood.

work against the depletion of platelets, and therefore solve only one of the blood cell problems.

When patients reach a dangerously low platelet count, their blood will not clot and they are at risk of bleeding to death. When this happens, the official guidelines from the American Society of Clinical Oncology (ASCO) recommend platelet transfusions and halting chemotherapy and radiotherapy, at least temporarily.[9]

Chemotherapy is normally given periodically in multiple cycles, and continues for many weeks. At the beginning of treatment, the time between cycles enables most patients to renew their population of platelets, usually in only a matter of days, before they undergo the next cycle of chemotherapy. As the treatment progresses the collapse in platelet number following each cycle of chemotherapy becomes more severe and the process of renewal takes longer. In patients who have undergone previous rounds of chemotherapy (whose bone marrow sites have often suffered permanent damage) the recovery of platelet count may take a considerable amount of time and may never occur at all.

Whenever a patient reaches that point and can't take chemotherapy anymore, it poses a major obstacle for the clinical oncologist, whose goal is to shrink the patient's tumor and slow the advance of cancer. Furthermore, patients with thrombocytopenia have poor prognoses of cancer survival, while consuming a lot of resources for supportive care and also experiencing potentially life-threatening complications from treatment.[10]

For all these reasons, the development of an agent able to support platelet production during cancer treatment would represent a major breakthrough. I decided to reach out to the doctor from CTCA that I had met at the trade show in Las Vegas. She remembered me clearly from our awkward encounter. Extremely courteous and true to her word, she quickly helped me set up an appointment with several top doctors at CTCA.

So here I was, a few weeks after that phone call, about to rent a car at O'Hare airport with Dr. Hall and drive fifty miles north of Chicago in heavy snowfall to "speak platelets" with a team at the CTCA Midwestern Regional Medical Center in Zion, Illinois.

I had sent ahead a complete file presenting my father's research on RNA fragments. I was eager to find out if a hospital system that prides itself on practicing an integrative approach to cancer care, supporting the patients physically and emotionally, would embrace the project. Or, would this institution reject the invention without even testing it—like the French medical establishment did—dubbing it as too "revolutionary."

Upon our arrival, we were given a brief welcome tour of the hospital, including the usual diagnostic and treatment suites, dining room, chapel, and library. It was impressive. I was surprised when I saw the large number of rooms dedicated to group activities, including a demonstration kitchen and even a party room. We were told that, indeed, CTCA cares about providing its patients with a more humane experience than the average hospital. It offers access to naturopathic doctors, acupuncturists and psychotherapists, along with the classic conventional treatments like surgery, chemotherapy, and radiation.

Seeing their commitment to their patients made me hopeful that the hospital management would be open to conducting a study on Beljanski's RNA fragments.

After the tour we were led into a small room where three people were waiting for us: Dr. James Grutsch, chief analytics officer for the hospital, Dr. Robert Levin, lead oncologist, and his nurse practitioner, Maryann Daehler.

It just so happened that Dr. Grustch, a tall, thin fellow with a dry sense of humor, had spent some time as a young researcher at the Pasteur Institute in Paris, France, and our connection was instantaneous.

As he recalled, "In those days, the Pasteur Institute was the leading institute of molecular biology in the non-English-speaking world. The French researchers were very driven, worked very hard, and were very competitive. I read Beljanski's work, and I thought about it. Beljanski was right on target. If he survived all those years under a director like Monod, who did not tolerate dummies, he must have been a darn good scientist. He had done all of the work to show us that we could potentially save lives with RNA."

Nurse Daehler, fitting her nurse title by exuding empathy and wholehearted attention to detail, said: "If these RNA fragments can indeed accelerate the replacement of platelets in patients undergoing very aggressive therapy for cancer, we ought to test them."

Dr. Levin, however, had serious reservations, "Why on earth would you invest in the study of a product which is already on the market? You should first study a product and only then put it on the market! This is going backwards!"

Dr. Hall explained that my father's pre-clinical studies were very promising and that the safety of the product had been well-established, but that no clinical trial had ever been conducted with it, and the effects on patients suffering from solid tumors were unknown. Chemotherapy drugs offered nowadays were different than those tested by Beljanski. He added, "We also need to know if the RNAs can raise platelet counts enough to make transfusion unnecessary—that would be a breakthrough. A clinical trial to test the RNA fragments in cancer patients undergoing chemotherapy will answer all these questions."

Dr. Levin seemed to remain hesitant, but Dr. Grutsch had all the right words, "RNAs are essential nutrients present in any diet.[11] The FDA looks at RNAs as food—so much so that baby formula manufacturers are now required to put both long and short chain RNAs in their products so babies have fewer rounds of diarrhea. This is something that the Institutional Review Board (IRB) of the hospital would like to see."

"This could potentially be very, very important," Nurse Daehler chimed in, pleading, "Don't we want to be the first to discover it and have it done here?"

All eyes were on Dr. Levin, who actually looked quite debonair with his salt-and-pepper locks and crisp white linen shirt.

"Fine. Let's test a dietary supplement. Nothing works for platelets so far, so I suppose we have to give these RNAs a chance," he concluded solemnly, as if it were history in the making.

I was beyond relieved: After having spent months vainly searching for a good, reliable source of Pao pereira, and tested—only to have to reject—dozens and dozens of samples, the interest of CTCA in the RNA fragments would now allow The Beljanski Foundation to move forward with a product that could be produced in quantity!

Because Beljanski's RNAs had never been tested in clinical conditions, we all agreed that the study should be designed to confirm the previous pre-clinical studies regarding the safety and the efficacy of the product. Dr. Levin and Dr. Grutsch suggested a trial design involving participants suffering from a range of advanced cancers including: breast, esophagus, nasopharynx, colon, and pancreas. All participants had been extensively pre-treated. Many had already failed multiple chemotherapies or were suffering from metastatic disease.

The patients would be administered a variety of chemotherapeutic drugs, including drugs known for inducing bone marrow suppression and thrombocytopenia. Eligibility for receiving RNA fragments was contingent on the potential onset of thrombocytopenia. The dose of RNA fragments would be escalated in 20 mg increments up to the maximum dose of 80 mg (20 mg, 40 mg, 60mg, and to 80mg) during the trial to provide some insight into what might be the best dose for an individual patient, and also allowing the doctors to monitor patients for any adverse effects.

I had two requests to make for the trial.

The first request was that patients should avoid taking benzodiazepine drugs while taking the RNA fragments. This was based on the notes of Dr. Marcowith.* Benzodiazepines are a class of psychoactive drugs commonly prescribed to treat insomnia and anxiety, which is why they are widely prescribed for cancer patients. According to Dr. Marcowith, benzodiazepines interfere with the RNA fragments and prevent them from working properly. Furthermore, according to a study released in the *British Medical Journal,* benzodiazepine use is associated with a significantly increased risk of developing Alzheimer's disease: those who took the cumulative equivalent of daily doses for three to six months over a five-year period were roughly 32 percent more likely to develop Alzheimer's than those who took none. Those who took the cumulative equivalent of a full daily dose for more than six months were 84 percent more likely to develop Alzheimer's.[12]

The market for sleeping pills and anti-anxiety drugs has exploded in the past several years, unfortunately with an associated explosion of Alzheimer's cases. The casualties can already be seen. According to the Alzheimer's Association, every 67 seconds someone in the United States develops Alzheimer's, and by mid-21st century someone in the United States will develop the disease every 33 seconds.

Dr. Levin balked at this first request. Many of his patients were indeed using benzodiazepines to fight some sort of depression. However, given that Dr. Marcowith had documented the possible interaction with the RNA fragments,* he agreed to defer to that finding and include the avoidance of benzodiazepines in the guidelines of the trial.

My second request concerned the Belgian-made yeast-based RNA fragments reported as non-effective at the New York symposium. I was hoping that they

---

*   See Bonus 1: Notes from Christian Marcowith, M.D.

could be tested as well, so that their effectiveness, or lack thereof, could be scientifically documented.

It was decided that the study would be divided in two. Thirty-two patients would receive Beljanski's E. coli K-12 based RNA fragments, and the same number of patients would receive the yeast-based RNA fragments. That would help determine if all RNA fragments are equally effective, or if the platelets activation was specific to Beljanski's E. coli K-12 RNA fragments.

This study on human subjects—the clinical trial at CTCA—was a significant achievement, even by my own self-effacing standards. I couldn't help wondering: *Am I done with fulfilling my promise to my father? May I now put this behind me and move on with my life?*

Those questions, as they flitted across my mind, brought with them a full range of emotions, and, finally, the realization that '*this*' had *become* my life. '*This*' was making me proud, and that pride had become essential for me. I was no longer merely carrying on my father's legacy. I was now proudly pursuing my own purpose, and I would not have it any other way. I was totally amazed at the transformation of my feelings—from the total rejection of my father's work as a young girl to the complete and proud acceptance of it as my very own.

But who said that following one's dream is a blissful experience, a revelation, a joyful ha-ha moment? For me, the shortage of *Pao pereira* had induced the highest level of stress. It turned the whole "realization and acceptance" thing upside down. *The dream I was following seemed rather to be a nightmare!* The shortage of botanical material was something that I took to heart as my personal failure, so much so that I could physically feel the onslaught of guilt and anxiety eating me alive and keeping me awake from dusk to dawn.

Research shows that when people are stressed, their bodies respond to physical, mental, or emotional pressure by activating the sympathetic nervous system, which releases stress hormones (such as cortisol, epinephrine and norepinephrine). These stress hormones increase blood pressure, speed up the heart rate, and raise blood sugar levels, all of which can improve our chances of survival in the event of high-stress situation that demands an immediate fight or flight response. Under chronic stress, however, the sympathetic nervous system is turned on virtually all the time. In this state, adrenaline and noradrenaline-stimulating mechanisms may very well end up altering the genetic code. That genetic alteration can lead to a number of pro-cancer processes, including the activation of inflammatory responses as well as the inhibition of immune responses and of the DNA-repair process.[13]

I was undoubtedly living evidence of the mind-body interaction. Totally sleep-deprived, I started to develop inflammation in my joints, and my hormonal imbalance was wreaking havoc. Determined to stay away from symptom-numbing medicine like steroids and anti-depressants, I tried stress release techniques like yoga, meditation, and acupuncture. Nonetheless, I remained a stressed-out ball of nerves.

Searching for support in the self-help section of Barnes and Noble, I stumbled upon *How to Stop Worrying and Start Living*,[14] a book by Dale Carnegie on tactics for liberating yourself from nagging anxieties. The book draws from the author's own experience as a struggling novelist. After two years of toiling away without much success, he decided to cut his losses and go back to teaching and nonfiction writing — which made him world famous.

He wrote, "After discovering the worst that could possibly happen and reconciling myself to accepting it, if necessary, an extremely important thing happened: I immediately relaxed and felt a sense of peace that I hadn't experienced in days," he wrote. His approach to any worry is a simple three-step plan: First, ask yourself what is the worst that could possibly happen; Second, prepare to accept the worst; Finally, figure out how to improve upon the worst, should it come to pass."

I sincerely tried. But I simply could not envision what the worst that could happen would look like. I could only acknowledge that my journey so far had been life-altering, and there was no way I could ever go back to practicing law. Trying to figure out what the worst could be and how to avoid it was impossible for me.

And yet, good things kept happening, despite my physical and mental distress.

I was introduced to Beth Barry, publisher at Demos Medical Publishing, a well-established company known for producing high-quality books for medical professionals. I immediately thought of my father's 1983 book, *The Regulation of DNA Replication and Transcription*,[15] originally published with Karger, but now out of print. In this book, Beljanski summarized his effort to identify the mechanisms responsible for the release of genetic information and their role in the regulation of cellular events.

Apart from its academic and historic significance, the book is a valuable resource on how to induce or control the expression of certain genes, and, moreover, to promote differentiation of given cells in vitro as well as in situ.

The publisher agreed to not only re-publish the book, but graciously went on to grant interviews* explaining her interest in Beljanski's visionary approach as the founder of "environmental medicine and integrative oncology."

Finally! I thought. *The mutation dogma laid down by Jacques Monod is no longer the reigning idea! Linking cancer to environmental health factors is now politically correct, and a new generation of scientists have understood and embraced the shift of paradigm!*

Around the same time, the Institutional Review Board at CTCA reviewed and approved the study protocol on RNA fragments and, once completed, the outcome of the clinical trial was published.[16]

First, the clinical trial concluded that Beljanski's E. coli K12 based RNA fragments (graciously provided by Natural Source International, Ltd.) were not associated with any negative side effects, and absolutely no toxicity was reported (even at the highest dosage of the fragments). In fact, many of the patients in the trial said they felt better while taking the product and others commented they even had more energy, despite their condition and their aggressive ongoing conventional treatments. Nine patients were treated with Carboplatin, ten with Adriamycin, nine with Cyclophosphamide, six with Cisplatin, eight with docetaxel, and eight with Mitomycin, which is known to be an especially aggressive chemotherapy. At all doses, patients receiving E. coli RNA fragments showed good recovery in platelet numbers, and none of the patients had an unplanned dose reduction or delay in their chemotherapy treatment. Finally, Beljanski's E. coli K12 based RNA fragments did not super-induce the numbers of white blood cells. Patients in the trial did not overproduce platelets; rather, these cells returned to normal range.

---

*   The movie "The Beljanski Legacy" is available on the YouTube channel of The Beljanski Foundation: https://www.youtube.com/watch?v=5dSz0bmwcj0

As Dr. Grutsch told *The Doctors' Prescription for Healthy Living* maga-zine, "This was a very exciting result. A natural product was helping our patients in a meaningful way to get through their chemotherapy. Many of these patients had failed several rounds of chemotherapy—we had some patients with ten or elev-en uncompleted cycles—and high doses of these RNA fragments appeared to be helping these patients complete therapy on time and without a reduction in their doses. They had all sorts of cancer—breast, pancreatic, colon, lung. The thing they had in common was that their chemotherapies were particularly aggressive—and with incredible failure rates. These were very challenging patients who had failed nine or ten earlier rounds."[17]

As for the patients using yeast RNA fragments, several failed to show any benefit at all.* We have all heard about the placebo effect—if you strongly believe something is going to help you, even a dummy sugar pill may often appear to help trigger some positive effect. But the yeast RNAs did not even provide that, as patients experienced dose reductions or delays in their chemotherapy treatment. Also, there was no evidence of any dose-response relationship between yeast RNA and platelet recovery levels.[16]*

E. coli K12 based RNA fragments are painstakingly long, difficult, and expensive to produce, but here was the scientific evidence that all RNAs are not created equal. One cannot cut corners—and costs—by using a cheap baker's yeast and expect similar results. I hoped that this publication[16] would provide people with further evidence that they should stay away from companies offering pale imitations of Beljanski's real products.

A battle had been won, but all the success surrounding the RNA fragments and publication could not steer me away from my haunting obsession with *Pao pereira*. It became overwhelming, almost suffocating at times.

I was deeply troubled. *What if the ongoing studies at Columbia University on Pao pereira demonstrate positive results on advanced prostate cancers that do not respond to hormonal treatments, and that revelation triggers a demand for the product that can't be fulfilled because of a lack of inventory? Is it ethical to raise people's hopes and then leave them high and dry? Or should I suppress the information, or at least delay it until the occurrence of a miracle in the form of several tons of tree bark?*

---

*   See Appendix 3: RNA Fragments comparison chart

Dr. Jun Yan was approaching the end of his fellowship with Dr. Katz's laboratory at Columbia University Medical Center. He had not completed the *Pao pereira* study, but he was so intrigued by the preliminary results that he was dedicated to continuing his research back home at the University of Nanjing, one of the oldest and most prestigious institutions in China. Dr. Jun Yan left the U.S. with the very last stash of powder, and then we waited for several agonizing months while he used the most up-to date techniques to determine how the *Pao pereira* extract exerts its effects, what molecules it influences in the cell, and what responses are triggered. Finally, his publication, "*Pao pereira* Extract Suppresses Castration Resistant Prostate Cancer Cell Growth, Survival and Invasion Through Inhibition of NFκB Signaling," came out in *Integrative Cancer Therapies,* a peer-reviewed quarterly journal focused on a comprehensive model of integrative cancer treatment.[18]

After the work done at Columbia with Dr. Katz had showed that *Pao pereira* inhibits the growth of prostate cancers that still respond to testosterone (LNCaP), the Nanjing study showed that it is also effective against the aggressive, drug resistant, androgen-independent PC3 prostate cancer cell line and, remarkably, the extract does so through several different biochemical pathways. Notably, the study revealed that *Pao pereira* acts on a signaling complex called NFκB—a control center regulating inflammation and cancer progression.

This finding brought to mind the fond memory of the elderly gentleman interviewed by Dr. Walker[19], who claimed his knees had improved while his prostate cancer had receded. I decided to send him a little note.

"Don't let anybody ever smile at your testimonial, or dismiss it as 'too good to be true'" I wrote. "There is a scientific explanation to your overall improvement: *Pao pereira* helps with inflammation!"

Men with advanced, metastatic prostate cancer, who were failing their hormonal treatment, had a new reason for hope!

If they could find some quality *Pao pereira* extract, that is.

Heartbroken, I decided to adopt a low profile with the publication, and delayed posting it on The Beljanski Foundation's website. What was I waiting for? A miracle.

And lo and behold, about a week later I received a call from the coffee grower's son in Cayenne, French Guiana. (I had not heard from him since the Heart of Palm Lady's drama.) He had a cousin in Argentina who was starting a new furniture manufacturing business and was in the process of importing various wood species. He was inquiring whether I would still be interested in—

"YES!" I don't think I even let him finish his sentence.

I wasted no time.

With a source of *Pao pereira* now secured, I was back in business, happily talking clinical trials with Dr. Katz. We agreed on conducting a small clinical trial on men with an elevated PSA (Prostate Specific Antigen) reading, giving them a combination of both *Pao pereira* and *Rauwolfia vomitoria*.

Interestingly, just like for men with advanced prostate cancer, there is not much currently offered to men with simply elevated PSA (averaging 8 to 10 on the PSA scale) as long as they have not been diagnosed with cancer. Our so-called "health system" is actually sick-centered. We don't do much for prevention, and even conveniently confuse the terms diagnosis and prevention. In fact, they are completely opposite: diagnosis is about recruiting more clients that will fuel the economy of the sick-centered system, while prevention is about *preventing* them from entering the system in the first place.

Millions of men have elevated PSA readings, with a negative biopsy. Dr. Katz was eager to see if *Pao pereira* and *Rauwolfia vomitoria* could help them. So Columbia University conducted a 42-patient study to confirm the absence of any safety concerns and to determine the best dosage of the extracts, which were offered as a special combination. All patients were supposed to have a negative biopsy before the trial in order to enroll, and then would have a second biopsy at the end of the trial in order to confirm the efficacy of the treatment. For the purpose of the study, patients were divided into groups of three.

The first group of patients each received two capsules daily of the combined herbs. Once they responded favorably, the next group was given three capsules.

Each subsequent group was given an additional capsule per day, and all the patients were followed for a twelve-month period.

We increased the dosage up to eight capsules a day, the maximum dosage we intended to try, and all patients responded quite well with no side effects reported. Although the safety of each ingredient had been previously well established, this clinical trial, though small, very effectively confirmed the safety of the combination.

Unfortunately, the study went too well from a scientific point of view. Many men, seeing their PSA level back to a normal range, decided not to undergo a second biopsy at the end of the study. With these opt-outs, Dr. Katz couldn't get the proper data he needed to publish. The study was incomplete, but certainly not in vain, as we learned that in addition to seeing a decrease in their PSA readings, men were reporting an improvement of the bladder issues that often come with prostate inflammation and enlargement.

For The Beljanski Foundation this was certainly a home run, since we now had gathered evidence through several separate studies that the same extracts could be useful on pre-cancerous cells, as well as regular cancer cells and advanced, metastasized, hormono-castration resistant, cancer cells. Melissa Burchill, a registered dietitian, summed it up in an article entitled "Two Herbal Extracts for Protecting Prostate Cell DNA."[20]

Dr. Katz was very happy with the results and gave a number of presentations later that year. In an interview with Dr. Coles for *The Doctor's Prescription for Healthy Living* he said: "We now know that this combination of Beljanski's extracts can significantly lower PSAs in a twelve-month period. Also, we have had very few patients convert to prostate cancer and have found a number of patients who have had a dramatic improvement in their urinary symptoms. Men are clearly having less frequency, better streams, and better flow rates. They are not getting up as often at night. The bottom line is that our early results are very encouraging regarding Beljanski's extracts' ability to lower PSA and also help older men urinate better."[21]

At one of Dr. Katz's lectures, I was approached by Dr. Jeanne Drisko, a professor at the University of Kansas Medical Center (KUMC) whose work on Vitamin C is internationally recognized. (Dr. Schachter had graciously introduced me to her at a previous ACAM conference.)

Dr. Drisko was very impressed with the results. "Wow!" she exclaimed, "This is fascinating. Do you have anything like that for women?'

"Yes." I replied matter-of-factly and without hesitation, "The same thing."

She reacted with an incredulous look on her face. I knew she was wondering how that could be possible. So I embarked, once again, on an explanation of how the extracts work at the level of the DNA by recognizing the destabilized DNA and blocking its duplication. This process makes the action of the extracts neither gender- nor organ-specific.

Breathlessly, she almost begged, "Do you think it could work on ovarian cancer?"

Ovarian cancer is one of the hardest cancers to address. First of all, there are often no obvious symptoms at its early stage, and the patient doesn't feel that anything is going seriously wrong. As a result, most ovarian cancers are diagnosed relatively late, which limits treatment options. Secondly, the tumor cells in ovarian cancers usually become resistant to the drugs chosen for treatment. The tumors may be reduced in the first stage of therapy, but when the cancer cells become resistant to the toxic effect of the drugs, they keep growing even in the presence of those drugs.

Another study with the botanicals? And for women, now!? How will I ever keep up with sourcing enough Pao pereira? My heart started pounding. But that didn't keep me from answering.

"Yes, definitely. According to his last publication, my father had positive results with his extracts on sixteen different lines of cancer cells, including ovarian cancer cells, so you should be at least able to confirm his work in vitro. It would also be most interesting to confirm the activity in vivo."

Dr. Drisko's big brown eyes suddenly seemed even bigger. She was looking at me like a kid looking inside a candy store!

"And what about pancreatic cancer?" she asked, "Do you think we can give it a try?"

I could hear the anxiety in her voice. Pancreatic cancer is a real monster. There are 32,000 people diagnosed each year in the U.S. alone, with a five-year survival rate of less than 5 percent after diagnosis.[22] Pancreatic cancer, just like ovarian cancer, is often diagnosed at a late stage, where the cancer is more advanced, and the tumor tends to become chemo-resistant. There is a compelling need for innovative treatments for both ovarian and pancreatic cancer, including an urgent need for agents that overcome the chemo-resistant characteristics of these tumors.

"I think it's worth giving it a try too," I heard myself say sheepishly.

And so began The Beljanski Foundation's collaboration with Dr. Drisko and Dr. Qi Chen at KUMC.

I should have been elated, but I was far too exhausted to feel happy about the new development.

Deep down, I had known for a while that I was in trouble. But I had dismissed the feeling. I was far too tired to even acknowledge it, much less address it.

CHAPTER NINE
A TOXIC WORLD

"A truly strong person does not need the approval of others any more than a lion needs the approval of sheep."

VERNON HOWARD

*O*ne of the main things I learned was that you could be doing all the right things and minding only your own business, and something totally outside your control could step in to cause catastrophe in your life. I also learned that recovery from that catastrophe can be devastating in and of itself and might lead to its own set of repercussions. Thirdly, and perhaps most importantly, I gained a better understanding of the phrase "Every cloud has a silver lining."

I had been dragging myself around for several months, battling an overall lingering feeling of exhaustion, along with chronic pain, dizziness, and headaches but had been postponing seriously addressing the issue for as long as possible.

I finally decided to get checked out. My doctor assured me that I was in "perfect health." I would've loved to believe it, but I couldn't. I was feeling more horrible with each passing day. I went to get a second opinion. That doctor said that if I felt tired I should take a vacation. In fact, he just happened to have a timeshare in Florida he wanted to sell.

A prescription for real estate? Seriously?!

Reluctantly, I went for a third and then a fourth opinion. Their conclusions were all the same: there was nothing wrong with me.

At some point, I decided that something was wrong with *them* if they couldn't provide me with a diagnosis that made sense!

I finally looked to the services of a kind and wise naturopath doctor in Long Island, who had me to take a simple urine test, which shortly thereafter revealed that I was "spilling arsenic." *Arsenic!* I was shocked. That sounded like a story for a film noir from another era! How could this be?

It turned out that heavy metal poisoning is more common than I had ever imagined. Metals like lead, mercury, cadmium, aluminum, and arsenic are all natural components of the earth's crust, and when the crust is disrupted by human activity, it can contribute to environmental contamination. Particles get dispersed by the wind, fall back to the ground, and infiltrate the soil, where they can remain for decades, poisoning water, crops, animals, and consequently the entire food chain. They can be found in the most unexpected places. Researchers at the University of California, Berkeley, tested various lipsticks (both drugstore and department store brands) and found that most contained high concentrations of titanium and aluminum. All examined products had detectable manganese, and lead was detected in twenty-four products (75 percent.)[1]

Mercury may already be in your mouth (amalgam fillings), as well as on your plate when you eat fish. Cadmium is everywhere: cigarette smoke, plastic packaging (where some leaches out into your food), cell phone batteries, and so much more. Arsenic is in water and may contaminate everything.

Heavy metals can enter the human body by way of food, water, air, or absorption through the skin. Even small quantities can be highly toxic, making it difficult to pinpoint one specific source, although rice is now said to contain more arsenic than any other cereal crop.[2]

Detoxification involves the removal of harmful toxins that build up in your body over time, especially in the liver, kidneys, lymphatic system, and colon. Normally the body takes care of its own detoxification process, but the production of industrial chemicals has risen rapidly since the Industrial Revolution, leaving us drowning in a sea of synthetics that find their way into the environment, and, ultimately, into living organisms.

The Mayo Clinic's website explains, "The liver normally removes and breaks down most drugs and chemicals from your bloodstream. Breaking down toxins creates byproducts that can damage the liver. Although the liver has a great capacity for regeneration, constant exposure to toxic substances can cause serious, sometimes irreversible harm."[3] Unlike the stomach, for example, the liver rarely tells you directly when it is upset. It will rather tell you indirectly by performing poorly, leading to toxin buildup that has been linked to a wide range of health problems, including developmental problems, heart disease, diabetes, and cancer.

Heavy metals in the human body have even been compared to enemy strongholds that suppress the immune system! My father published on the topic, showing that the destabilization of DNA can be triggered by heavy metals.[4] Moreover, it is also said that as those heavy metals accumulate in those loops specific to destabilized DNA, each metallic molecule acts like a mini antenna that is interfering with our electromagnetic fields, thus increasing the risk of inducing cancer.

I wasn't there yet, but I also learned that we are not all equally equipped for coping with pollution, and that I have a slight genetic liver deficiency, making it harder for my body to process and eliminate the constant onslaught of toxins. I had no choice but to flush out the poison through intravenous Chelation Therapy (IV).

Chelation therapy consists of a series of intravenous injections (usually anywhere from ten to fifty) of a synthetic amino acid solution—EDTA (ethylenediaminetetraacetic acid)—into the bloodstream. The word "chelate" comes from Latin "chela" and Greek "khele," which both mean "claw." The solution "grabs" the heavy metals and helps eliminate them from the body through the kidneys.

Chelation therapy was created almost by accident in the early 1930s, when Ferdinand Munz, a German chemist, was looking to create a new water softener. It proved to be particularly effective in treating lead poisoning, and was largely used in the 1950s to treat workers who had painted U.S. naval vessels during World War II with lead-based paints.[5] But in the 1960s the collusion between money and power led, once again, to the suppression of a useful therapy. EDTA fell into disrepute, and only a few doctors since have been performing chelation. Few doctors even test their patients for heavy metals. Dr. Garry Gordon, who sits on the Board of Homeopathic Medical Examiners for Arizona and is co-founder of ACAM explained the following in a 1997 exclusive interview granted to *Life Enhancement* magazine[6]:

"In 1966 or 1967 the American Medical Association ("AMA") Special Division of Occupational Medicine held a high-level meeting. AMA came out of this meeting with a statement saying it was virtually malpractice for doctors to prescribe oral EDTA. The reason they did it was basically because doctors paid by the lead industry had some guidelines put together by the Occupational and Health Boards of the U.S. government stating that you could keep people on the job even if their blood lead level was as high as 60 or 80 μg/dL. Now we know blood lead is unsafe at a level as low as 10 μg/dL."

Despite its well-documented safety and efficacy, EDTA chelation therapy has remained the subject of a smear campaign by the governmental/medical/pharmaceutical complex.

I went through seventeen weekly sessions of intravenous chelation therapy, sitting in the same treatment room with patients receiving chemotherapy. Most offered small, compassionate smiles toward the newcomer. Some looked at my hair with envy. Until then, it had never occurred to me that my modest mane could inspire envy.

Rubber band, needle, and drip, drip, drip...for fifty minutes or so. Silence reigned, inviting each of us to meditate on his or her own mortality.

I bruise easily, and soon my arms were covered with marks. I quickly became self-conscious about my arms, constantly hiding my needle tracks with long sleeves as if I were a drug addict. A worse side effect was that the intense detoxification process wiped out what little energy I had left, at least for the first ten sessions. Driving back home after each session was a difficult—and somewhat dangerous—experience. Once, as I pulled over for a few minutes to rest my head on the steering wheel, I remember thinking: *If I am genetically wired to be a sponge for arsenic, it is only a matter of time before it starts accumulating again. There must be a better way than going through this cycle again and again!*

For people who are only mildly poisoned with heavy metals, and for those who have already addressed their acute state of heavy metal toxicity, oral chelation is an option. But the chelating agent EDTA is very poorly absorbed by mouth (only about five percent is absorbed). The unabsorbed 95 percent of EDTA remains within the digestive tract where it mixes with undigested food. In the long term it may prevent the normal absorption of such essential minerals as zinc, manganese, chromium, vanadium, copper, chromium, and molybdenum. In turn, that potentially leads to nutritional deficiencies, possibly worsening the very problems supposedly being treated. (DMSA, another chelating agent, has difficulty crossing the human blood–brain barrier. That limits its use to extracting heavy metals from parts of the body other than the central nervous system, which poses a different problem altogether.)

The IV chelation worked remarkably well for me. It proved extremely helpful with getting rid of my arsenic intoxication, and had no other side effects besides the extreme exhaustion in the early stage of the treatment. However, I was certainly not excited about fighting chemical poisoning with the ingestion of even more chemicals. I felt there should be another way—a gentler, natural way—for combating heavy metal poisoning as a chronic issue.

During the following weeks, I searched various health food stores and pharmacies, but couldn't find anything close to what I had in mind. I was looking for a product that would encompass each essential step of supporting the liver's effort to flush out toxins: the capturing of the heavy metals, the binding to the proper substrate of fibers, and finally allowing for the all-important elimination process. Otherwise, toxins will be "recycled" by the body and re-absorbed.

Suddenly, a larger vision dawned on me. Since my father's philosophy was based on the idea that environmental toxins destabilize DNA, a comprehensive and holistic "Beljanski Approach to Wellness" should encompass the avoidance of toxins to the fullest possible extent. It should further help remove the toxins that we already have in our bodies, and support and rejuvenate the functioning of the body's systems through potent and complete whole-food formulas, providing a superior source of vitamins and minerals, plus a wide array of antioxidant protection.

Research soon convinced me that this Approach to Wellness could and should be seen as a must by everyone. A study spearheaded by the Environmental Working Group (EWG) found an average of 200 industrial chemicals and pollutants in umbilical cord blood from babies. Tests revealed as many as 287 chemicals in umbilical cord blood, 180 of which are known to cause cancer in humans or animals, 217 of which are toxic to the brain and nervous system, and 208 that cause birth defects or abnormal development in animal tests.[7]

And that's just for starters.

As soon as we begin eating and drinking as young children, additional sources of pollution find their way into our bodies. In 2012, the U.S. Food and Drug Administration (FDA) banned Bisphenol A (BPA)—a chemical commonly used for decades in polycarbonate plastic products and epoxy resin-based food can liners to harden plastic, keep bacteria out of food, and prevent rust—from being used in the manufacturing of all baby bottles and sippy cups. However, many consumer products, such as food storage containers, plastic tableware, and food packaging, are still manufactured with BPA. Animal studies show that BPA mimics the hormone estrogen and disrupts the natural balance of the endocrine system. Even low levels of BPA affect the hormones that control the development of the brain, the reproductive system, and the immune system. In laboratory rats, exposure to BPA has been linked to an increased risk of some cancers, decreased sperm counts, reduced fertility, and hyperactivity. The National Institutes of Health (NIH) and the Environmental Protection Agency brought together experts who reviewed seven hundred studies published on BPA. They found that the BPA levels in humans are typically higher than the levels causing adverse effects in animal studies.[8]

Consider a life-long exposure to numerous chemicals and pesticides, heavy metals, and the daily lathering with all the expensive preservatives, dyes, and fragrances contained in our luxury hygiene or beauty products,[9] and you will understand why Mirko Beljanski was a visionary when he suggested that cancer could result from the progressive and cumulative destabilization of DNA.

Striving for the removal of toxins is a necessary first step towards good health. Unless someone considers living in a bubble, the removal of toxins is a must. Then, supporting and rejuvenating the functioning of the body's own systems through potent and complete whole-food formulas, providing it with a superior source of vitamins and minerals, plus a wide array of antioxidant protection, is the necessary next step to protect our health. (There is a significant difference between natural and synthetic vitamins: natural vitamins come with various bioflavonoids, those cofactors thought to increase the bioavailability of vitamins by 30 percent. Synthetic vitamins, on the other hand, contain no cofactors, and research suggests that they can even deplete the existing resources in the body, eventually causing vitamin and cofactor deficiencies).

Finally, the obvious last step of the Beljanski Approach to Wellness should be to counteract the damage already done, and use the extracts *Pao pereira* and *Rauwolfia vomitoria* that block the duplication of destabilized DNA!

I pledged to myself that if I ever get better, I will create a line of products that will help eliminate toxins and provide quality support to the body's rejuvenating process.

And I am going to start using some Pao pereira and Rauwolfia vomitoria extract right away, preventively, to fight the possible damage arsenic may have already done to my body. *

Having made that decision, I started to feel better.

I soon received comforting news from Kansas.

At KUMC, Drs. Chen and Drisko, recognizing that "natural products have long been proven a considerable resource for bioactive anticancer agents,"[10] had been evaluating the antitumor effects of both *Pao pereira* and *Rauwolfia vomitoria* extracts in various pancreatic and ovarian cancers, two notoriously difficult cancers to treat. Although current chemotherapy can improve the five-year survival rate, it has not increased the overall rate of cure. 70 percent of patients experience a relapse and develop a resistance to platinum- and taxane-based treatments; malignant ascites (a fluid buildup in the abdominal cavity) happen quite often, causing extreme discomfort while the survival rate plummets to a crushing 5 percent.

In light of such horrendous statistics, patients and their families often question the value of conventional treatments, but are not quite sure what alternative regimens there are to follow. They are under pressure to make life and death decisions. Everybody in the family has an opinion, emotions fly high, and often families (and even couples) get torn apart at a time where unity and support are most needed.

---

*   Visit www.beljanski.org to learn more about the Beljanski Approach to Wellness.

Under such circumstances, a synergistic action between conventional chemotherapy and a natural supplement taken orally, one that would allow the reduction of the toxic burden of the former and at the same time enhance the benefits of the overall treatment, seemed an appealing goal to the Kansas team. They also intended to research whether the natural extracts would be able to continue exhibiting proper anticancer activity by themselves in the face of drug resistance, which is a very common and devastating issue that leaves doctors at a loss for therapeutic options.

The first round of study was *in vitro*. Five pancreatic and three ovarian cancer cell lines were tested, and both extracts were selectively active against those cancer cells. To test whether the extracts could enhance the cancer cells' sensitivities to chemotherapy drugs, they were combined with Gemcitabine to kill pancreatic cancer cells and Carboplatin to kill ovarian cancer cells. Both combined treatments significantly enhanced cell death in cancer cells that were strongly resistant to the drugs—which was exactly what the Kansas team was hoping to see.

After reviewing Dr. Chen's data, Dr. Hall noted, "If this translates into animal studies, we will have not one, but two winners!"

We didn't have to wait long.

Drs. Chen and Drisko were just as excited as we were. Soon after those initial results, they injected several groups of mice with drug resistant pancreatic or ovarian cancer cells, and then treated them. At optimal doses, tumor growth was significantly suppressed by both extracts alone. When combined with chemotherapy drugs, both extracts remarkably enhanced the effect of the drugs and the reduction of the tumor burden.

In ovarian cancer, when *Pao pereira* and Carboplatin were used together in the animals, the tumors decreased by a whopping 82 percent.[10] The *Pao pereira* also helped decrease the volume of malignant ascites by 55 percent on its own, and eliminated ascites completely when combined with Carboplatin (a major achievement, considering the severe health complications induced by the ascites). The same happened with the *Rauwolfia vomitoria*: tumor growth in mice, treated with the botanical alone, was suppressed to a degree comparable to that of Carboplatin alone. The volume of fluid from ascites and the number of non-blood cells in those ascites were also significantly decreased. When the *Rauwolfia* extract was combined with Carboplatin, it remarkably enhanced the effect of Carboplatin and reduced tumor burden by 87 percent to 90 percent and ascites volume by 89 percent to 97 percent.[11]

Just as with ovarian cancer, the scientists were able to confirm the tumor inhibitory effect of the *Rauwolfia* either alone or in combination with Gemcitabine for pancreatic cancer. The synergy of action was also confirmed: notably two mice in the "Gemcitabine plus *Rauwolfia vomitoria*" group experienced complete tumor regression, an effect that was not observed in any other treatment group. "As Gemcitabine alone did not provide any benefit in inhibiting metastasis, *Rauwolfia*, or Gemcitabine plus *Rauwolfia* combinations, significantly improved the effect versus Gemcitabine alone."[12]

Finally, I believe the *Pao pereira* paper on pancreatic cancer[13] brought a smile to Dr. Dale O'Brien's face. Dr. O'Brien, an Assistant Clinical Professor at the University of California at Davis in the Department of Medicine, is also Executive Director of Cancer Patients Alliance and the Medical Director of the alliance's Pancreatica and CancerPACT projects. He has been an affiliate of the European Branch of the World Health Organization and of the Epidemic Intelligence Service of the Centers for Disease Control and Prevention (CDC).

Dr. O'Brien dedicated a blog entry on the Pancreatica website to the results of the latest study:

"The current study is somewhat elaborate. The *Pao* showed inhibition of all five of the pancreatic cancer cell lines that were studied. Also, the combination of *Pao pereira* plus Gemcitabine showed synergy in the inhibition of these cancer cell lines. Finally, *Pao pereira* and Gemcitabine alone and in combination were presented to live mice with pancreatic cancer tumors (PANC-1) which were then serially scanned. The *Pao pereira* showed significant action in inhibiting tumor growth. And the combination of *Pao pereira* coupled with Gemcitabine showed even more apparent activity (inhibition). This is the kind of serious science that we love to see with alternative therapies. It appears at this early stage that *Pao pereira* is worthy of further study – possibly eventually making its way to clinical trials. There are many stages to this of course, but this research is a refreshing clean look at an interesting, potentially effective, new treatment agent for the treatment of pancreatic cancer."[14]

I wrote back on my blog,* to express my appreciation. I was seeing a brilliant future for the research. I was seeing easier funding. The satisfaction, however, did not last long. One morning, I woke up in a pool of my own blood. I had had a long history of ovarian cysts and fibroids, but I had never reflected on it, until then.

My parents had devoted their lives to studying the effect of molecules on other molecules. In their home, either because of modesty or coldness, emotions were deemed "inappropriate." Isn't it ironic how our educational system is all about mathematics and literature, while so little is done to prepare our children for life's real challenges, which always revolve around the handling of strong emotions?

Despite my family's disdain for everything not scientifically established, I have always been intuitively convinced that we are much more than a simple bunch of molecules: thus my interest in body-mind connection. This intuition of mine was reinforced by listening to cancer survivors' stories. Their testimonials brought upbeat reports about their recovery once they started taking the extracts, but I was mostly interested in asking questions about their circumstances at the time of the occurrence of the disease. Those questions almost always opened the door to a story of personal dramas involving relatives, ranging from devastatingly painful losses to conflicts with toxic people.

"Toxic people" are the people who might resent your progress for any number of reasons. Falling short of controlling their own lives, they try to control yours. They will take pleasure in telling you, in more or less subtle ways, that you are not enough. They tell you these things until you give up and take the guilt message to heart, where it will slowly poison you.

Looking back, many long-term cancer survivors declared cancer as the silver lining that allowed them to reset their emotional counter and reinvent a healthier life for themselves.

I had a great interest in Dr. Ryke Geerd Hamer's approach to disease, and the link he proposed between specific emotions and the organs where cancer would

---

* www.thebeljanskiblog.com

subsequently arise. On August 18, 1978, when Dr. Hamer was head internist in the oncology clinic at the University of Munich, he received the shocking news that his son, Dirk, had been shot. Dirk died four months later, and several months after his death, Dr. Hamer was diagnosed with testicular cancer. He wondered if his son's death could have triggered his cancer.

Dr. Hamer subsequently investigated and documented over fifteen thousand cases of cancer and found the disease to always be linked to an emotion (e.g. anger, frustration, grief) that affects us on three levels: psyche, brain, and a specific organ linked to the trauma by subconscious association. According to Hamer, the cause of cancer is a traumatic experience for which we are emotionally unprepared. The brain will start sending wrong information to the organs it controls, resulting in the creation of deformed cells in the tissues: cancer cells.

The implication, that solving an emotional conflict is the first step to healing the disease, did not sit well with the official cancer establishment, which makes its living by recommending drugs, surgeries, and conventional treatments. As a result, Dr. Hamer was jailed.

Today, however, the link between cancer and emotions has been largely accepted. As the saying goes, "Give it time and the truth will surface."

In her book *Molecules of Emotion,* neuroscientist Dr. Candance B. Pert writes, "We can no longer think of the emotions as having less validity than physical substance, but instead must see them as cellular signals that are involved in the process of translating information into physical reality, literally transforming mind into matter. Emotions are at the nexus between matter and mind."[15]

It thus makes sense to look at negative emotions as another layer of the "stuff" that could contribute to the destabilization of DNA. A big emotional shock may very well be the culprit that will, in some people, precipitate the cancer phenomenon. There is no doubt in my mind that negative emotions must be dealt with as an integral part of understanding the root of a disease and its cure, and that the proper approach to disease is neither entirely psychological, nor solely physiological. However, inasmuch as I was intellectually interested in understanding how it worked with others, I wasn't ready to do the work for myself.

Through my research, I stumbled onto the description of the personality traits of the cancer-susceptible individual, especially well-described by Dr.

Douglas Brodie, Director of the Puna Wai Ora Mind-Body Cancer Clinic in Taumarunui, New Zealand:

> "In dealing with many thousands of cancer patients over the past twenty-eight years, it has been my observation that there are certain personality traits present in the cancer-susceptible individual. These traits are as follows:

1. Being highly conscientious, caring, dutiful, responsible, hard-working, and usually of above average intelligence.

2. Exhibits a strong tendency toward carrying other people's burdens and taking of extra obligations, often "worrying for others."

3. Having a deep-seated need to make others happy. Being a "people pleaser" with a great need for approval.

4. Often lacking closeness with one or both parents, which sometimes, later in life, results in lack of closeness with spouse or others who would normally be close.

5. Harbours long-suppressed toxic emotions, such as anger, resentment and / or hostility. The cancer-susceptible individual typically internalizes such emotions and has great difficulty expressing them.

6. Reacts adversely to stress, and often becomes unable to cope adequately with such stress. Usually experiences an especially damaging event about two years before the onset of detectable cancer. The patient is not able to cope with this traumatic event or series of events, which comes as a "last straw" on top of years of suppressed reactions to stress.

7. Has an inability to resolve deep-seated emotional conflicts, usually beginning in childhood, often even unaware of their presence. Typical of the cancer-susceptible personality, as noted above, is the long-standing tendency to suppress "toxic emotions," particularly anger."[16]

I recognized that many of the above traits applied to me, and that I had done nothing to uncover—much less address—my own emotions. Instead, I had buried them for a long time under a frantic pace of activity. I had proudly rebranded my denial as "having faith in the universe" and a belief that "everything will work out in the end."

I woke up in a hospital bed, exhausted and feeling utterly defeated. Earlier that morning, when I discovered I was bleeding, I knew I had no choice but to call for an ambulance and surrender to hospital care. Immediate surgery to remove my uterus, cervix, and ovaries had been presented to me as the only option.

Soon after I emerged from the anesthesia, a nurse entered and told me I was very lucky. My tumor was benign. As she left, I distinctly heard the same little inner voice that had told me again and again to chin up and carry on: *You are lucky.... this time!*

A shiver went through my spine.

Was this a warning from beyond? A sign to be deciphered? Could it be that the heavy metal chelation had reduced the toxic load in a timely fashion to protect me? Had the six capsules of *Pao pereira* and *Rauwolfia vomitoria* I had been swallowing daily for weeks prevent any bad cells from multiplying?

I lay staring up at the ceiling, my mind empty. And then, perhaps because the anesthesia had inhibited my usual suppression mechanism, a question popped forcefully into my mind: *AND NOW WHAT?*

The nurse reentered, giving me a reprieve from the battle raging in my mind.

I glanced at the tray she had brought me: a bowl of macaroni and cheese, along with a glass of orange juice obviously poured from concentrate. My brain immediately started to assess the meal before me: lactose, sugar, preservatives, additives and gluten (most likely from wheat spread with the carcinogenic pesticide glyphosate.) My stomach churned. If food is our medicine, as Hippocrates said, I knew right away this particular food was going to be bad medicine for me. It almost always requires a progressive and cumulative combination of several factors to destabilize the DNA and trigger cancer. Not only will sugar fuel cancer cells, but a diet too high in sugar and protein will modify the normal flora of the intestine and induce the development of a pathogenic putrefactive flora, which will poison the organism at several subtle levels. A primal connection exists between our brain and our gut, which contains a hundred million neurons that watch over our digestive well-being, including the way we "digest" our emotions.[17]

The time had come to say, "No."

I was hooked to several tubes and my ability to move was quite limited. But I managed to turn my head to inspect the space surrounding me and discovered that

I was alone. I had a long look at the empty chair next to my hospital bed, the empty bed next to mine, and allowed the realization to set in. I don't know what would've happened if some other patient had been lying in the other bed, distracting me from taking in the deep feeling of loneliness, but also of peace and quiet. At that moment, I realized that I had been repeatedly ignoring the signals sent by my body for years. I finally acknowledged that the troubles with my female organs were just the reflection of my own conflicted emotions as a woman.

Suddenly, to my drugged mind, everything became crystal clear and oh so simple: the chair next to my bed was empty because my husband wasn't there for me. I had allowed myself to marry a man who was emotionally unavailable, just like my own father had been. Neither of them had been bad persons, but although their paths, circumstances, and personalities were otherwise completely different, both had proven unable, for their own reasons, to provide me with the attention and affection I had been craving.

With that realization, an earthquake occurred within me, creating a brutal shift of emotions. And then, all the sudden, it was over. After all those years of pining away within myself, I was done. Done longing for closeness and seeking validation from an outside source. Done cherishing the wait. Done longing for an embrace that was not meant to be. I had finally arrived at the doorstep of reality. No anger. No resentment. Just plainly done. And I was ready. Ready to hold myself accountable for not seeing the truth before the "I do's" had been pronounced, and for entering a relationship that was doomed to be unfulfilling.

Forgiving myself proved to be more difficult. Deep down something kept screaming that I should've known better. Nevertheless, I reasoned that drumming up the culpability card was not going to help me answer the big question: *AND NOW WHAT?*

I was finally free from a lifetime of frustration and ready to run with my life... as soon as I could run!

Convinced that the tumor on my uterus, although fortunately benign, was a symptom of "dis-ease" that I could no longer ignore, I knew that being true to myself was the only way to make peace with the past and move forward towards a physically and emotionally healthy life.

It was there, in that small bed at Lenox Hill hospital, that I resolved to file for divorce.

CHAPTER TEN
A UNIQUE UNDERTAKING

"Aggressive therapies are used when a Doctor is not skilled
enough to make the most of gentle therapies."

DR. ISAAC ELIAS

W*e are not all alike. Nor do we all face the same challenges in life.
Nor do we have the same dreams. But each of us has a unique purpose, an inner calling, a reason for being on this earth. Finding this
purpose may not come easy. Doubtless, many have gone on without
this knowledge in their possession. But once you find it, it's like finding a GPS
that will keep you on track towards your true destiny.*

According to the American Cancer Society, the number of cancer cases
around the world is expected to double by 2030. An aging population, combined with increased pollution, and global access to weapons of mass destruction in the form of pre-packaged foods and sugary drinks, have created the
"perfect cancer storm."

Where shall we run for safety?

Mirko Beljanski's extracts are not going to offer a global solution: definitively, there would not be enough raw material. But Beljanski offered the
world a new vision of cancer that should open the door to new and exciting
avenues of research for a young generation of scientists. Far ahead of his time,

he looked for progressive and cumulative destabilization of DNA as the root cause of cancer while his peers were looking for mutations. That led him to create his own unique test of carcinogenicity: the Oncotest, which measures the degree of DNA destabilization induced by certain products and materials. The test allowed him to make the breakthrough discoveries of anticancer molecules in natural extracts, molecules that were selectively toxic only to cancerous or pre-cancerous cells.

The good news is that we now know that such molecules exist! As they selectively kill many kinds of cancer cells (including cancer stem cells), they are non-toxic to healthy cells, and work in synergy with most chemotherapies.

The bad news is that this is not where pharmaceutical companies are investing their money.

Whatever their differences, health care systems around the world are all plagued by ever-increasing costs and long waits at hospitals for expensive conventional treatment. Some systems work better than others in terms of reimbursements, accessibility, and coverage, but they are all straining under the pressure of spiraling cost and reduced access.

One would think that if there were evidence of a product or treatment that could begin to address these problems, it would be embraced by mainstream science and the politicians in charge of our future.

Think again.

With cancer being a multi-billion dollar per year business, it's no surprise that pharmaceutical companies will protect their brands at all costs and decry natural solutions as quackery, even if this blanket rejection of natural treatments screams conflict of interest. The industry warns that if natural treatments are allowed to flourish, "Desperately ill patients clinging to false hope may refuse surgery or give up their medicine and die." Meanwhile, the industry continues to treat only the symptoms—the consequences of the sickness and not the cause of sickness — while imposing ever higher prices on its products.

My father was a casualty of this corrupted and compromised system. I get it.

What I was not prepared to experience was the long-lasting hatred beyond the grave. Two decades after his passing, there are media companies that continue to spend time and energy promoting negative views on the Internet of Beljanski's research, and of Beljanski personally.

Who is still paying them?

On February 14, 2013, at lunchtime, a French TV channel (France 5) presented an "informational" program about Mirko Beljanski, entitled "Hero or Crook?" The presenter dismissed Beljanski's work by claiming he hadn't shared his results! It was an obvious lie, considering that Beljanski left a legacy of 133 scientific publications, two books, and eleven patents to protect and therefore describe, his products. When The Beljanski Foundation requested an opportunity to reply and set the record straight, France 5 rejected the request.

I beg to ask the question: what on earth is strong enough to motivate a TV channel to use its prime time on Valentine's Day to trash the memory of a scientist who passed away some fifteen years earlier?

Some governments have even taken the fight against Beljanski's scientific achievements a step further, by prohibiting their own people from accessing the natural molecules he discovered. In a memo dated January 1, 2013, the Belgian *Agence Fédérale des Médicaments et des Produits de Santé* stated, "*Pau pereira* (*Geissospermum*) is not characterized well enough to ensure quality and safety of commercial preparations,"[1] lending its legal authority to a national prohibition against sale and distribution of the product.

This is especially ironic considering that 19th century medical authorities in Belgium were promoting the use of *Pao pereira* as a "new remedy" to fight tropical fevers. In 1887, *Le Journal de Médecine, de Chirurgie et de Phamacologie*, published in "Nouveaux Remèdes" ("New Remedies") the following note: "Pereirine (the old name for flavopereirine, *Pao pereira*'s active ingredient) would be more effective than quinine against malarial fevers. The dose of 2 g of hydrochloride is to be taken four hours prior the access."[2]

Similarly, it was in Belgium that the first modern chemical characterization of *Pao pereira* took place, when, in 1959, Puisieux published an article on the nature of some of the alkaloids from *Geissospermum*![3]

There are only two logical explanations for Belgium's reversal of scientific opinions: either science has been going backwards in Belgium since the nineteenth century, or the 2013 decision from the *Agence Fédérale des Médicaments et des Produits de Santé* was entirely political.

Benjamin Rush, one of the Founding Fathers of the U.S. and a signer of the Declaration of Independence, was already promoting public health by advocating medical freedom in the 18th century:

> "Unless we put medical freedom into the Constitution, the time will come when medicine will organize into an undercover dictatorship to restrict the art of healing to one class of Men and deny equal privileges to others; the Constitution of the Republic should make a special privilege for medical freedoms as well as religious freedom."[4]

Unfortunately, the Founding Fathers did not take Rush's advice. Medical freedom was not included in the U.S. Constitution, and now we are faced with a corrupted, drowning health system. There is no more dire or prophetic depiction of this state of affairs than what bestselling author Dr. Ghislaine Lanctôt wrote in the introduction for the 2002 re-edition of her book *The Medical Mafia.*[5]

> "Competition is being eliminated. Researchers are being reoriented. Dissidents are imprisoned or being shown up and reduced to silence. The alternative products that are profitable are being recuperated by multinationals thanks to the legislation of the Codex of the WHO (World Health Organization) and the patents of the WTO.
>
> Cunningly stoked by the authorities and the media that serves them, a fearful panic of sickness, of aging and of death is haunting the population. The obsession to survive at all costs makes the international traffic of organs, blood and human fetuses prosper...also at all costs.
>
> Food is irradiated, milk pasteurized, genes modified, water is contaminated, and the air is poisoned. Children receive thirty-five vaccines before entering the school system. Whole families are drugged; the father on Viagra, the mother on Prozac, and the children on Ritalin. Soon, their security, their normality, and their happiness will be assured by the implantation of the microchip, as we do with animals. Infertility clinics will produce, by artificial insemination, triplets and quadruplets, and a good quantity of embryos are being stockpiled. Human cloning is around the corner. You have gone mad."

We do not want to go mad. Most of us simply want the safest, most effective option available, whether it's food, herbs, or a pharmaceutical drug. And for those who have been told their condition is terminal, alternative medicine may offer precious hope they thought was lost. But choosing between herbs and drugs is often difficult because the information that we need to make these decisions is largely unavailable. There are two reasons for that. The first one is purely economic and has nothing to do with the effectiveness of natural compounds: pharmaceutical and biotech companies invest heavily to create new-to-nature molecules they can easily patent, in order to create lucrative monopolies.* That is why there is very little money and interest from the pharmaceutical companies for natural compounds (but plenty for "analogs"). The second reason is regulatory: not only is little money invested in research with natural compounds, but herb and supplement manufacturers who dare research their products can be put out of business if their research is deemed by authorities to reveal an *intent* of bringing to market a product that could help treat a medical condition. One would think that there could be no serious objection to accurately informing the public about any lawful activity. After all, the First Amendment requires liberty to discuss publicly all matters of public concern. But since the enactment of the Dietary Supplement Health Safety Act in 1994, manufacturers making health-related claims or deemed to make an implied claim, or even deemed to have the intent to make a possible claim on food products, have been prosecuted.

The First Amendment is the cornerstone of all our individual rights, and that is precisely why it came first. It has been successfully used again and again to limit the intrusion of government and to prohibit many forms of censorship. It has even been successfully invoked to prevent the government from restricting the dubious political activism of those "super PACs" able to buy their way into the election process.

---

* The U.S. Patent and Trademark Office (USPTO) asserts that natural products no longer can be patented because of the Supreme Court's 2013 decision in *Association for Molecular Pathology v Myriad Genetics,* in which the court ruled that the isolation of genes that are found in nature does not make them patentable. On March 4, 2015, the USPTO updated its guidelines for patent examiners, instructing them to reject patent claims that seek to protect all purified natural products, not just DNA. This new guideline makes patenting extracts of natural products even more problematic than in the past, and some patent attorneys question whether paclitaxel would be approved today.

Source: Hirshfeld AH. "2014 procedure for subject matter eligibility analysis of claims reciting or involving laws of nature/natural principles, natural phenomena, and/or natural products [memorandum]." *United States Patent and Trademark Office.* March 4, 2014.

"When Government seeks to use its full power, including the criminal law, to command where a person may get his or her information or what distrusted source he or she may not hear, it uses censorship to control thought. This is unlawful. The First Amendment confirms the freedom to think for ourselves."

Citizens United vs. Fed. Election Com'n, 130 S.Ct. 908 (2010)

Incredible as it may seem, the principles articulated by the Supreme Court in this case have not been extended to supplement manufacturers.

Originally, the hardline approach against supplements was developed to protect a largely uneducated public against 19th century snake oil traveling salesmen like William Avery Rockefeller, (1810-1906, and yes, the father of John D. Rockefeller). He was selling a cure-all tonic he called "Rock Oil" and charged $25 a bottle for it, then the equivalent of two months' salary for the average American worker. "Rock Oil" was in fact just a mixture of laxative and petroleum and had none of its various claimed benefits. Rockefeller, however, never stayed in one place for very long, so he didn't have to worry about the consequences when his customers discovered they'd been had.

The days of William Avery Rockefeller are long gone. In the age of the Internet, any law aimed at protecting a naïve public is clearly outdated. However, disclosure about the benefits of a dietary supplement or food, no matter how credible and documented, places it in the category of "unapproved drugs." The American Association for Health Freedom (AAHF) states, "The FDA ignores first amendment protections and censors the communication of valid scientific information. The agency seems to have lost sight of its mandate to protect the public and has instead come to see itself as the guardian of corporate interests."[6]

If "Ignorance leads to the loss of Freedom," as Benjamin Franklin has taught us, there is no doubt that the intent of this policy is to keep us ignorant and deprived of our freedom of choice.

To add insult to injury, since 1983 when Boots aired the first broadcast television commercial in the United States for the pain reliever Rufen, pharmaceutical companies have been allowed to place ads on television.[7] Every few minutes, on every TV set, in every American living room, the same scenario is playing again and again: a reasonably attractive and easy-to-identify-with model will suffer from a litany of symptoms until popping a pill. Within a matter of seconds, bye-bye frowning, hello smile. The promise is always the same: "Ask your doctor for this prescription drug and you will get your life back."

If it sounds too good to be true, it probably is. According to a 2013 report on nightly news broadcast slots on the U.S. East Coast between 2008 and 2010,[8] 57 percent of the most emphasized claims in prescription and non-prescription drug commercials were found to be potentially misleading. A further 10 percent were demonstrably false or unsubstantiated by publicly available evidence. And yet, no matter how false and obtrusive, these marketing messages have delivered billions to pharmaceutical companies, while generating a giant epidemic of prescription drug abuse all over America.

To put an end to this nonsense (and obvious double standard with respect to the First Amendment), a bi-partisan bill, the "Free Speech About Science Act," was introduced to Congress on April 5, 2011.

What could be wrong with pushing for quality research and transparency? Which congressman would vote against that?

As David Steinman, publisher of *The Doctor's Prescription for Healthy Living*, put it, "By considering complementary and alternative medicine (CAM) therapies that have been proven in the laboratory and in clinical trials to offer benefits to cancer patients with no toxicity, clinicians are able to offer more options to their patients and improve their overall care."[9]

Many consumers are looking for reliable information backed by legitimate scientific research to assist them in making informed choices. But for the deep pockets who have long enjoyed their monopoly upon free speech, allowing dietary supplement manufacturers to promote scientific evidence, however truthful, did not seem like a good idea. Not surprisingly, the "Free Speech About Science Act" quietly died in some House Committee in Congress soon after its introduction. It never made it to the floor of the House, and our representatives never had a chance to vote on it.

In 2004, *Fortune* magazine dedicated a full issue to cancer research. On the cover, in capital letters was the question: "Why We're Losing the War On Cancer?"

Under this provocative title the intriguing tagline appeared in parentheses: "And How to Win it."[10]

Clifton Leaf, the article's author listed a number of "miracles cures that weren't," including radiation therapy, Interferon, Interleukin-2, Endostatin, and Gleevec. He concluded that we need to "change the way we think about cancer" and went on to quote Eli Lilly's Homer Pearce:

"I think everyone believes that at the end of the day, cancer is going to be treated with multiple targeted agents—maybe in combination with traditional chemotherapy drugs, maybe not. Because that's where the biology is leading us, it's a future that we have to embrace—though it will definitely require different models of cooperation."

That is exactly the approach Mirko Beljanski developed—but with natural molecules.

As journalist Michele Cagan wrote in a newsletter for the *Health Sciences Institute Members Alert*:

"Dr. Mirko Beljanski took a view of cancer that no one had ever seen before. When he looked at carcinogens (substances that stimulate cancer cells but not healthy cells), he realized that there must be some substances that act in the opposite way—substances that would destabilize cancer cells, but leave healthy cells alone [...] With this brilliant new concept, Beljanski tried to change the way we treat cancer patients. That was more than twenty years ago, and the mainstream still hasn't caught on."[11]

And until the mainstream catches on, this wealth of knowledge will not be secured, despite the best efforts of The Beljanski Foundation.

How can we make certain that this body of work is not again at risk of disappearing?

One way is by each of us making it our duty to reach out to as many people as possible and share this life-saving information. We will take back our power over health, and exercise our sovereignty by promoting the funding and sharing of scientific information that has the potential to disrupt a societal order that continues to kill us.

Every time you see a conventional doctor, ask questions on prevention, nutrition, and lifestyle. Tell your doctor that you expect him or her to take the time to get to know you and discuss your health goals. A quote attributed to Hippocrates says, "It is more important to know what kind of person has a disease, than to know what kind of disease a person has."

We have a right to self-determination. You may ask your doctor what the alternatives are to conventional treatment. Your doctor should assist you with reviewing all the options that science offers. Ask your doctor for a synergy of action between natural and conventional treatment to reduce the toxicity associated with chemotherapy. If your doctor says that such a thing does not exist, give him or her a copy of this book.

Ask how normal cells will be protected from the side effects of your treatment. Ask explicitly how the removing or killing of cancer cells will affect normal cells. If the doctor measures success by the size of the tumor with CT scans or PET scans and offers a chemotherapy treatment, ask for studies showing an overall improvement of length and quality of life. According to the final results of a large, randomized clinical trial presented at the 2008 annual meeting of the American Society of Clinical Oncology (ASCO), patients who received the chemotherapy drug Gemcitabine after surgery for pancreatic cancer lived two months longer than patients who had surgery alone.[12]

Ask about cancer stem cells, those 1 percent to 5 percent of cancer cells that will resist conventional treatment and can metastasize. If cancer stem cells resist chemotherapy and radiation, what will destroy them? Ask about the foreseeable consequences of killing "regular" cancer cells, while leaving out cancer stem cells. Doing so merely kills their competition and allows them to flourish.

Ask your doctor how to protect your healthy tissues during radiotherapy, and how to maintain your platelets during chemotherapy. If you are advised not to take supplements during chemo or radiation treatments, be specific and ask your doctor for scientific evidence of any negative effects of those supplements when taken with these therapies.

Tell your doctor that you don't want to take a chance on a therapy that may fail you, and ask for "personalized medicine." While the tailoring of treatment to patients is just good practice and dates back at least to the time of Hippocrates,[13] the term is now fashionable in medical circles due to new fancy diagnostic and informatics tools. The Research Genetic Cancer Center (RGCC) is a genetic research laboratory that operates globally, while headquartered in Greece. RGCC has developed a patented membrane that is able to capture malignant cells from a simple blood sample. Then they match those malignant cells recovered from the blood sample with a panel of known anticancer agents and see what will indeed work. No more guessing, no more false hope. Originally created to allow oncologists to select the chemotherapy treatment that would be the most effective against each specific cancer, it also allows other practitioners to know what may be the best natural approach to cancer therapy. In Japan, where the test is routinely prescribed, a specific mix of *Pao pereira*, *Rauwolfia vomitoria*, and golden *Ginkgo* extracts has been confirmed as having the ability to induce apoptosis (death) of the cancer cells for many patients suffering from different cancer types. A Japanese doctor has been kind enough to share with The Beljanski Foundation his data on 40 patients.*

As for the extracts themselves, I cannot stress enough the importance of the quality of the natural extracts being used. Obviously, only quality extracts sufficiently loaded with active ingredients will trigger an apoptosis of cancer cells. Beware of the inconsistency in potency from one brand to another. There can be a huge difference in concentration between various extracts available on the market, as shown in a comparative study conducted by an independent laboratory commissioned by The Beljanski Foundation.**

Beware also of substances only backed by unverified testimonials. Look instead for compounds where the mechanisms of actions have been studied and published in reputable scientific journals (for example, Columbia University's experiments showing that *Pao pereira* induces apoptosis, or *Rauwolfia vomitoria* induces cell-cycle arrest, two well-documented ways to effectively kill cancer cells). When you find such a study, check for the name of the company listed as the source of the compound which has been tested. Don't buy from copycats. More

---

*   Learn more on www.beljanski.org

**   See Appendix 2: Pao pereira content comparison chart (Flavopereirine)

often than not, cheap imitators "borrow" the science made by serious companies and present the results as if obtained by their own product. They will sell you snake oil medicine (Rockefeller style) swearing it's the same or even better than the original. Look for the trademark. Serious, quality products are trademarked. The trademark should appear visibly on the label. Only one company has been authorized to use the Beljanski trademark, and the products it sells are the same quality as the ones being used for research.

Finally, expect that your approach will be resisted, not only by conventional doctors, but also by large nonprofit organizations that are cozy with the mainstream. This has been my personal experience. One would think that a large, highly regarded foundation whose mission is "to advance the scientific and medical research related to the diagnosis, treatment and cure of pancreatic cancer" (according to its website) would take a serious interest after receiving an article entitled, "Inhibition of Pancreatic Cancer and Potentiation of Gemcitabine Effects by the Extract of *Pao pereira*" published in *Oncology Reports Journal*,[14] as well as another article, "Antitumor Activities of *Rauwolfia vomitoria* Extract and Potentiation of Gemcitabine Effects Against Pancreatic Cancer" in *Integrative Cancer Therapy*.[15]

Well, no, not at all.

Instead, the big foundation politely indicated that it wasn't interested in helping The Beljanski Foundation fund the next round of research.

At first, I was floored: *They are not interested in learning more? Seriously?* A non-toxic compound with a selective action against cancer cells, and exhibiting an excellent synergistic action with Gemcitabine chemotherapy, is by every standard a scientific breakthrough.

But then I realized that this rich foundation wasn't going to put its money into something that has not received the blessing of pharmaceutical companies, and pharmaceutical companies are solely looking for corporate profits that only synthetic molecules can yield.

Next time you're solicited by a charity to fund research, ask what the money they collected last year was specifically used for, and ask if there is any scientific publication to show for it. I've been surprised to find how many people don't think to ask how their money is used.

How many billions of dollars have been spent in vain on the war on cancer since President Nixon signed the National Cancer Act of 1971?

As long as the pharmaceutical companies' quest for innovation is solely driven by intellectual property rights,[16] they will keep failing in the war on cancer. This intellectually reductive approach prevents most scientists from looking in the right places to treat cancer. In the face of this failure, those who are supposed to be accountable for our malfunctioning public health policies will instead witch hunt the free thinkers and discoverers who dare defy the laws of money, think outside the box, and, in the end, offer substantial help to humanity.

The good news is that more and more good doctors are refusing to be turned into five-minute prescription dispensers. They recognize that medicine is a holistic, multifaceted discipline. They value nutrition, psychology, and environmental medicine as part of their medical practices. Meanwhile, patients are becoming more and more empowered and educated. In growing numbers, patients are seeking new personalized solutions to replace the old one-size-fits-all approach to medicine.

Over the years I have seen many great individuals courageously and relentlessly fight their cancers—and win. All of them have prevailed by taking control of their lives, and making sure that "they never, never, never give up," as Sir Winston Churchill, an expert at winning war, once advised.

In this context, I strongly believe that the work done today by The Beljanski Foundation is of utmost importance. First, because of the scarcity of quality research on natural compounds, and, second, because of the importance of Beljanski's contribution to the advancement of science. At the theoretical level, Mirko Beljanski's discovery of the destabilizing role of environmental toxins to the DNA—that is to say at the very core of our cells—is central to understanding carcinogenesis. At the practical level, his ideas were validated by the development of products that have yielded astonishing good results for several decades and offer new and promising avenues of research.

Since 1999, The Beljanski Foundation, a New York City-based 501(c)(3) nonprofit organization, has sponsored research on the anticancer properties of the extracts discovered by Dr. Beljanski. These research programs, conducted with several high-profile institutions, have all led to many peer-reviewed publications.

The work done by the Foundation has enabled those institutions to confirm that two of the natural molecules discovered by Beljanski:

- Are selectively active on many kinds of cancer (including prostate, ovaries, pancreas)

- Help with precancerous cells (like elevated PSA levels)

- Are effective on cancers that no longer respond to chemotherapy

- Work in synergy with many chemotherapy drugs, all without side effects

- Work against cancer stem cells.

Additionally, a clinical trial confirmed the efficacy of another of Dr. Beljanski's discoveries for maintaining a healthy level of platelets during chemotherapy treatment.

In 2016, The Beljanski Foundation held a symposium in New York City to look back on the road traveled over the past twenty years since the French Army raided Beljanski's laboratory and put an end to his research. Doctors and scientists who have worked on the various research programs were there to present their results,* and many more came to support the Foundation through their generous donations. As I am writing these lines, new and exciting results are in the pipeline.

I do believe that there is a tipping point. If enough people choose a natural way to fight back against the disease, the economics currently driving the War on Cancer will eventually change. We are at the forefront of a Natural Revolution. The scientific rationale has been established. One day, maybe soon, the laws will change and it will make economic sense for companies to turn to Nature to cure cancer the natural way.

My father used to say, "When we have the power to help, we have the duty of doing so." Nothing makes me happier than sharing his powerful legacy of hope. I always had an inkling that the potential of what I was serving was much bigger

---

*   Interviews available on www.beljanski.org

than what I was going through, but I had no idea how lucky I was to be given the opportunity to make my life so meaningful. As a lawyer, I certainly didn't need to get involved in this adventure. But in the end, I'm so glad I did. Far from the rejection I felt as a little girl, today whenever I hear a great testimonial to my father's products, I feel grateful.

And now, my dear reader, the duty is yours to share this life saving information. It is up you to help make a difference in the War on Cancer—the natural way. A lot has been accomplished, many milestones have been achieved, but there is still much to do.

EPILOGUE
THE TEA ROUTE—
HOMECOMING

"Listen to the wind, it talks.
Listen to the silence, it speaks.
Listen to your heart, it knows."

NATIVE AMERICAN PROVERB

I n 1985, Professor M.C. Niu, head of a beautiful and brand new Biology Institute in Beijing, China, was facing quite an unusual problem. Professor Niu had been able to modify the tail of a fish by using the RNA of another fish from a different species, but he couldn't isolate the famous Reverse Transcriptase enzyme that would explain how he did it.

Beljanski's landmark discovery of the Reverse Transcriptase in bacteria had finally been published, both in French[1] and English,[2] despite all of Monod's efforts at the Pasteur Institute to bury it. Professor Niu was intrigued. He was hoping to show the existence of this enzyme in fish eggs, but so far, he hadn't been able to find any trace of it. He finally invited my parents to come to Beijing and work with him on researching the famous enzyme in fish eggs.

Beljanski was eager to confirm the importance of Reverse Transcriptase with a new study, as it would open new perspectives for understanding evolution. It was also a great opportunity for my parents to escape the suffocating atmosphere of the Pasteur Institute. Beljanski and Niu established a life-long relationship based on mutual respect. As for the goldfish eggs, it turned out that Beljanski thought of adding a drop of blood (rich in iron), and soon, they could evidence how RNA was able to carry the genetic information. That discovery led to a shared publication that reflected the results of their collaboration.[3]

Professor Niu wouldn't let my parents leave China without a ceremonial gift: a large sample box filled with China's finest teas. At the time, tea was already associated with valuable antioxidant properties, but Beljanski was determined to test his samples for specific anticancer properties.

Back in his laboratory, Beljanski subjected each sample tea to his famous Oncotest. He wrote down the results on a single sheet of paper, then filed the paper in a drawer, where it remained for several years.

In 1996, when Beljanski's laboratory was ransacked by the French army, all the cabinets and drawers were forced open and their contents were turned upside down. A truckload worth of documents was seized and whatever did not fit in the truck was abandoned, scattered all over the floor. A few days later, Gilda, his long-time assistant, walked to the laboratory to assess the situation and bring back some order to what looked like a crime scene (which in many ways it was). At her feet, literally, she found a piece of paper, bearing what she immediately recognized as my father's handwriting. It was a list of various kinds of teas, and, next to four of them the mention, "very anti-C." She sent me the paper, just in case it might be of value.

I located an organic source for each of the four teas, then blended them together.

As I sat quietly in the silent room to pour myself a cup of tea, I chose a nice, delicate cup of thin porcelain, one that would allow the soothing warmth of the cup to gently heal my worn hands. I directed all my attention to the golden liquid as it flowed out of the teapot into the tea cup. I looked at this cup of tea as if it was the center of my entire universe, then closed my eyes, inhaled the subtle scent, and allowed my mind to quiet.

Holding the cup with both hands, I marveled at how one's mind, heart, and hands may supernaturally align to design destiny. I swallowed a sip of tea, and welcomed the peaceful joy that results from feeling as if you have finally come home.

Maison, I thought, and smiled.

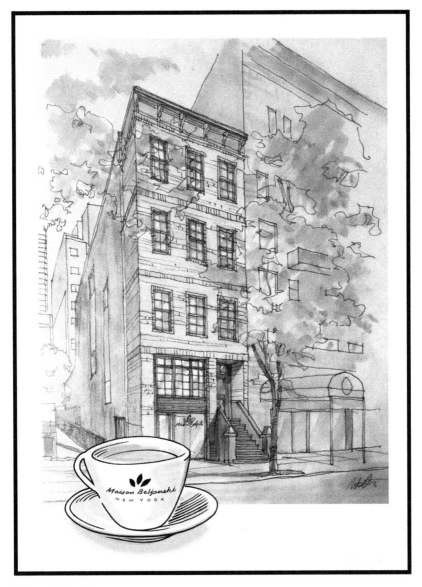

Maison Beljanski.

BONUS

Bonus 1: Notes from CHRISTIAN MARCOWITH, M.D.

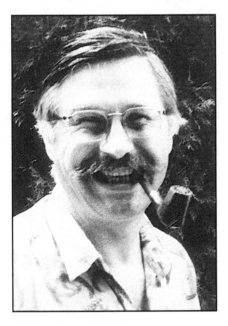

Christian Marcowith, M.D.

Christian Marcowith, MD, was a well-regarded family doctor who maintained his practice in a little village in Burgundy, France. Curious and open minded, he was always on the lookout for the best solutions for his patients. When Dr. Marcowith met Mirko Beljanski, PhD, the two started a conversation that continued until Marcowith's passing in 1996.

In a notebook assigned for the use of Dr. Beljanski, Dr. Marcowith suggested dosage amounts for each of Beljanski's discoveries, as well as treatment details that he found effective. The information is invaluable for physicians prescribing Beljanski's extracts for patients suffering from any form of cancer or from other degenerative diseases such as hepatitis, herpes, HIV, prostatitis, and many more.

Ms. Marcowith has generously bequeathed to The Beljanski Foundation all rights to her husband's notebooks. Dr. Marcowith's notes have been translated and reproduced here, with The Beljanski Foundation's permission.

Christian Marcowith, MD, was a well-regarded family doctor who maintained his practice in a little village in Burgundy, France. Curious and open minded, he was always on the lookout for the best solutions for his patients. When Dr. Marcowith met Mirko Beljanski, PhD, the two started a conversation that continued until Marcowith's passing in 1996.

In a notebook assigned for the use of Dr. Beljanski, Dr. Marcowith suggested dosage amounts for each of Beljanski's discoveries, as well as treatment details that he found effective. The information is invaluable for physicians prescribing Beljanski's extracts for patients suffering from any form of cancer or from other degenerative diseases such as hepatitis, herpes, HIV, prostatitis, and many more.

Ms. Marcowith has generously bequeathed to The Beljanski Foundation all rights to her husband's notebooks. Dr. Marcowith's notes have been translated and reproduced here, with The Beljanski Foundation's permission.

There are two main anticancer botanicals: ***Pao pereira*** **and** ***Rauwolfia vomitoria***. Both kill cancer cells and only cancer cells. They have no toxic effect on the individual. They are taken orally; if possible they should be swallowed several times throughout the day with meals. As they do not have the same target in the cell, taking them together doubles the individual's chance of destroying cancer cells.

Both can be used alone as a preventative measure or as a treatment; however, it is important to understand that these two products work in synergy with conventional treatments, meaning that each one maintains its individual mode of action, but the therapeutic effects are compounded.

Pao pereira fights cancer cells with no side effects. It can be used either as a treatment or as a preventative measure. In addition, the alkaloid in this herb can cross the blood-brain barrier which makes it possible to add it to any treatment protocol for brain cancers and certain viruses. Still, in the latter cases the dose of *Pao pereira* must be increased since only a small fraction of the product crosses the meningeal barrier.

Other than its anticancer activity, *Pao pereira* is a strong inhibitor of viruses, including viruses with RNA genomes (such as influenza, HIV, FEV (feline), hepatitis C, etc.) as well as DNA genome viruses (such as hepatitis A and B and herpes). *Pao pereira*'s effectiveness is not affected by hormones.

Rauwolfia vomitoria also fights cancer but with a special affinity for hormonally-dependent tissues, including the breast, prostate, testes, thyroid, uterus, ovaries, cervix, etc. Thus, this remedy is very desirable if the organ affected is hormonally-dependent. *Rauwolfia vomitoria* can be taken to combat the negative effects of menopause, or as a preventative measure in the case of suspicion or risk of a particular pathology. *Rauwolfia vomitoria* does not have any anti-viral effect and does not cross the blood-brain barrier.

RNA fragments from Escherichia coli K-12 bacteria do not work as an anticancer agent or as an antiviral agent. Instead, the small fragments of RNA, from Escherichia coli K-12, are used to stimulate the generation of immune cells and platelets (thrombocytes), which helps patients to better protect themselves from infection. In a situation where conventional cytotoxic therapies (chemotherapy, radiation therapy, and surgery) have been received, the RNA fragments protect the patients' physiology from the harsh effects of these treatments.

In older people, natural immunity has a tendency to diminish, so the ingestion of one dose per week of small RNA fragments is advised as a preventative measure. One dose is also advised for those people undergoing diagnostic X-ray examinations, vaccinations, etc., which are able to suppress the immune system.

For many autoimmune diseases, there is immunological disorder; therefore, ingesting a few doses of E. coli RNA fragments can be quite beneficial. These RNA fragments are taken orally and should be dissolved or melted in the mouth without water. Avoid the use of benzodiazepines when taking RNA fragments.

Beljanski's *Ginkgo biloba* is unlike any other conventional *Ginkgo biloba* extract, and so is its application. Beljanski's unique *Ginkgo biloba* extract is made exclusively out of golden leaves subjected to a very specific extraction process. Beljanski's *Ginkgo* extract is highly recommended for anyone undergoing anticancer treatment because disease coupled with conventional treatments works to disrupt normal protein functioning, which poses a danger for the patient. Additionally, certain diseases may cause protein buildup, one of the many cancer markers, for example, as well as other cancer markers like gamma GT and transaminases. The golden *Ginkgo biloba* extract can significantly help control this process of cancer marker production. In addition, it protects against fibrosis which is often induced by radiation over time, as well as the burns that may accompany radiation treatment.

Without exhibiting any detrimental side effects, the particular extract of *Ginkgo biloba* developed by Beljanski has proven beneficial to nearly all patients.

Protocol for Breast, Prostate, and Uterine Cancers

These endocrine system tumors affect organs that secrete specific hormones or growth factors. The protocol for these types of cancer are as follows:

Pao pereira: 4 to 5 capsules per day

Rauwolfia vomitoria: 4 to 5 capsules three times per day 20 to 30 minutes before each meal.

Golden leaf *Ginkgo biloba*: 4 to 6 capsules per day

RNA fragments from Escherichia coli: should be taken if the white blood cell and platelet counts are low due to radiation or chemotherapy treatments. In this case, start administering the RNA fragments the day before any cytotoxic treatments begin.

The RNA fragments, which come in the form of powder, should be held sublingually (under the tongue) until dissolved, 2 to 3 times per week on an empty stomach. Avoid drinking liquids immediately afterwards. Test the patient's blood count often.

Protocol for Thyroid Cancer

Pao pereira: 6 to 8 capsules per day

Rauwolfia vomitoria: 4 capsules per day

Golden leaf *Ginkgo biloba*: 4 capsules per day

RNA fragments: to be taken according to results of the blood cell count test

Protocol for Skin Cancer

Pao pereira: 6 to 8 capsules per day

Rauwolfia vomitoria: 4 capsules per day

Golden leaf *Ginkgo biloba*: 4 to 6 capsules per day

Protocol for Carcinoid Tumors in the Small Intestine

In addition to conventional radiation or chemotherapy treatments, take:

Pao pereira: 4 to 8 capsules according to the severity of the case

Rauwolfia vomitoria: 4 to 6 capsules per day

Golden leaf *Ginkgo biloba*: 4 capsules per day (especially if undergoing radiation)

Protocol for Tumors of the Large Intestine

Due to a strong hormonal response, the risk of intestinal cancer is greatly increased in people with thyroid problems.

In addition to conventional treatment (preferably radiation therapy), take:

Pao pereira: 8 to 10 capsules per day during aggressive treatment; 6 to 8 capsules thereafter

Rauwolfia vomitoria: 4 to 6 capsules per day

Golden leaf *Ginkgo biloba*: 4 capsules per day

RNA fragments: 2 or 3 doses a week in the event of aplasia (defective cell count)

Protocol for Esophageal and/or Stomach Cancer

In addition to regular, conventional cytotoxic or radiation treatment, the cancer patient may greatly benefit by taking:

Pao pereira: 6 to 10 capsules per day during aggressive treatment; thereafter reduce to a maintenance dose of 4 to 6 capsules daily

Rauwolfia vomitoria: 3 to 4 capsules per day

Golden leaf *Ginkgo biloba*: 4 to 5 capsules per day

RNA fragments: to be added if the patient experiences a reduced level of white blood cells or platelets

Protocol for Pancreatic Cancer

This is an extremely difficult malignancy to overcome. In addition to conventional treatments (generally radiation therapy and/or chemotherapy) take:

Pao pereira: 10 capsules or more each day

Rauwolfia vomitoria: 5 capsules per day

Golden leaf *Ginkgo biloba*: 6 to 8 capsules per day

Monitor transaminase and gamma GT, which are cancer markers indicating the cancer's evolution.

Protocol for Brain Tumors

In addition to radiation therapy, the cancer patient may benefit from the fact that the active ingredient in the *Pao pereira* extract crosses the meningeal barrier and shows a synergy of action with radiation therapy that fights brain cancers. *Pao pereira*'s antiviral action will allow it to fight certain viruses which induce brain cancers.

Pao pereira: 8 to 12 capsules per day

Golden leaf *Ginkgo biloba*: 4 to 6 capsules per day (especially in the case of radiation therapy to help avoid the fibrosis caused by radiation waves)

Protocols for Myeloma and Leukemia

A three-pronged approach may be advantageous in the case of myeloma or leukemia:

A – *Pao pereira* extract acts in synergy with conventional treatments to strengthen the inhibition of malignant cells and/or the inhibition of viruses, which are known to often play a role in the formation of malignant hemopathies.

For the aggressive phase: 2 *Pao pereira* capsules per 22 lbs. of body weight per day (approximately). Then reduce the dosage to 1 capsule per 22 lbs. of body weight per day (approximately). Capsules should be taken before breakfast and dinner.

B – RNA fragments preserve normal bone marrow cell replication and, therefore, stimulate immunity: 1 dose every other day during chemotherapy and 2 doses per week outside of treatments.

The number of platelets must also be monitored each week and dosage increased if necessary (maximum: 3 doses per week).

If aplasia is required (as in the case of bone marrow transplants) do not administer RNA fragments.

Ferritin, a protein that stores iron, forms as a result of the damage caused to erythrocytes (red blood cells) by chemotherapy. Some chemotherapy drugs enter the bone marrow, mainly in the liver and spleen, and prevent the formation of red blood cells. Humans need 2.7 million red blood cells per microliter of blood to ensure sufficient oxygenation (for syntheses) and to ensure that RNA fragments can work effectively. However, when RNA fragments are given to a patient with low red blood cell counts, it may help them avoid complications. The medical technician can do a red blood cell transfusion and then give the RNA fragments, which should immediately start to work; one will then note the increase in leucocytes (white blood cells) and platelets.

The addition of magnesium makes it possible to reduce the activity of the excess of ribonucleases in the patient's plasma.

Cytotoxic agents used for chemotherapy are invariably accompanied by unwanted adverse side effects. For instance, response to chemotherapy is very often accompanied by malignant cell resistance and resistance of certain enzymatic dysfunctions. In these cases, one particular Beljanski remedy works well. It is:

C – Golden leaf *Ginkgo biloba* helps to regulate the activity of numerous enzymes. The administration of this herb is straightforward: 2 capsules of Dr. Beljanski's unique *Ginkgo* extract in the morning and evening starting at the beginning of chemotherapy treatment.

Protocol for Bone Cancer

Bones afflicted by cancerous tumors lose calcium and phosphate. These two minerals tend to form a combined coating which covers the tumor and protects it against the effects of the natural extracts. However, after cauterization with radiation, the tumor will once again be treatable.

Pao pereira: 8 to 10 capsules per day

Golden leaf *Ginkgo biloba*: 4 capsules per day

RNA fragments: should be taken during radiation therapy

Protocols for Lymphoma Cancers

A – Skin Lymphoma

Pao pereira: 3 capsules morning and evening, 20 minutes before mealtime

Rauwolfia vomitoria: 2 to 3 capsules per day (as much for its cumulative effect as for its florescent marker effect and also because this anticancer remedy has to do with hormonally dependent tissues by means of testosterone)

B – Non-Hodgkin's Lymphoma

Pao pereira: 8 to 10 capsules per day (during aggressive treatment with radiation therapy)

Golden leaf *Ginkgo biloba*: 4 to 6 capsules per day

RNA fragments: to be adjusted according to blood cell levels

C – Hodgkin's lymphoma

Pao pereira: 8 to 10 capsules per day

Golden leaf *Ginkgo biloba*: 4 to 6 capsules per day

IDEAL DURATION OF TREATMENT WITH DR. BELJANSKI'S PRODUCTS

Pao pereira **and** *Rauwolfia vomitoria*: take these two inhibitor extracts together for their synergistic effect.

a. Start as early as possible following diagnosis.

b. Take the supplements over the course of the day, before breakfast and dinner.

c. Continue, concurrent with other traditional therapies, until the clinical state has once again become satisfactory. To be prudent, the patient may continue with extracts for a month or two past this point.

d. Later, engage in cyclical usage for preventative purposes for 2 to 5 months per year.

RNA fragments:

Start just after chemotherapy or radiation treatments have begun when they are inducing a drop in white blood cells (unless aplasia is the objective). Continue until white blood cells and platelets have returned to normal. Take one dose, sublingually, 1 to 3 times per week. Do not drink any liquid immediately afterward. Ideally the RNA fragments should be dissolved under the tongue on an empty stomach.

If the patient is taking heparin: ingest RNA fragments either twelve hours before or twelve hours after use of this drug.

Golden leaf *Ginkgo biloba*:

In order to regulate or curb hyperactivity of certain enzymes, use this herb in synergy with traditional cytotoxic treatments. For radiation burns, begin use just before ionizing treatments are received; continue until the end of radiation treatments, and for up to a month afterwards. Previous fibroses may also be treated. The sooner the herb is given, the better the results.

CANCER PREVENTION

Pao pereira and *Rauwolfia vomitoria* extracts have no side effects and the body does not develop resistance to their healing effects. In the absence of cancerous cells to attach themselves to, the molecules of alkaloid present within the two herbs (the actual healing agents) are rapidly eliminated from the body since they only bond with deregulated cells. Consequently, these extracts can easily be taken as a means of prevention in all precancerous states. They can also be used in recurrent cycles as a means of prevention for people with a high risk of developing cancer.

RNA fragments, in the same way, can be ingested with no toxicity as a means of prevention or repair for chromosomal breakage that inevitably accompanies the ionizing radiation in diagnostic tests (mammography, scintigraphy, X-rays, etc.). Take one cone-shaped unit of RNA fragments 24 hours before the examination and another one day after.

Bonus 2: Claim your complimentary access to
an on-demand CME credit webinar.

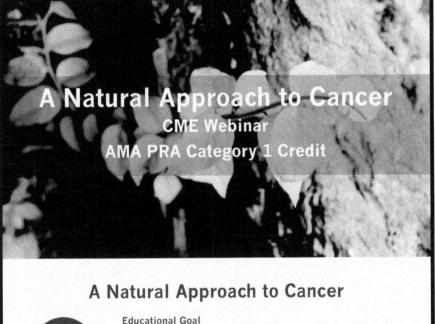

A Natural Approach to Cancer

Educational Goal

The goal of this activity is to enable the learner to explain the prevalence and health problems associated with environmental toxins and the theory of DNA destabilization from those toxins.

Learning Objectives

Explain the destabilizing effect environmental toxins have on the physical structure of DNA.

Describe the mechanism of action of natural non-toxic substances that work at the DNA level (which are not organ or gender specific) to selectively block duplication of cancer cells.

CME

Check our website and register now to attend

the online and on demand CME webinar

THE *Beljanski* FOUNDATION
A 501(c)(3) nonprofit organization

www.beljanski.org

WEBINAR: A NATURAL APPROACH TO CANCER
A ONE-HOUR CME WEBINAR PRESENTATION PROVIDING AMA PRA CATEGORY 1 CREDIT™

The Beljanski Foundation is pleased to provide AMA-accredited Continuing Medical Education for U.S. integrative healthcare professionals. *A Natural Approach to Cancer* is a one-hour CME webinar presentation with specific learning objectives that provides AMA PRA Category 1 Credit™ – the highest continuing education accreditation available for licensed health professionals in the U.S.

A Natural Approach to Cancer explores the underlying scientific theories and breakthroughs on DNA destabilization made at the Pasteur Institute by famed molecular biologist Mirko Beljanski, PhD, and recent validating research programs conducted at Columbia University, University of Kansas Medical Center, and other prestigious U.S. medical institutions. The presentation will also cover Dr. Beljanski's discovery of and clinical studies of natural extracts that act at the cellular level selectively on destabilized DNA.

As a bonus for purchasing the book, you are able to access the link three times. This program is not sharable. After you complete the webinar you will be able to download your Certificate of Completion.

To redeem your complementary access:

1. Visit http://shop.beljanski.org/cme/continuing-medical-education.html

2. Add the webinar to your cart

3. At checkout, enter the code: WEBWINWAR

4. Visit The E-learning tab on your account

5. Access the CME

6. If you are a healthcare professional, you will be able to download and print the AMA PRA Certificate after completion of the webinar.

APPENDICES

Appendix 1: **Scientific Publications of MIRKO BELJANSKI**

1. A propos du microdosage du ribose dans les acides nucléiques et leurs dérivés :
   a) M. BELJANSKI, M. MACHEBOEUF, C.R. Soc. Biol. 1949, CXLIII, pp.174-175.
   b) M. BELJANSKI, Ann. Inst. Pasteur, 1949, 76, pp. 451-455.

2. F. GROS, M. BELJANSKI, M. MACHEBOEUF, F. GRUMBACH, « Comparaison biochimique d'une souche bactérienne sensible à la streptomycine avec une souche resistante de même espèce. » C.R. Acad. Sci., 1950, 230, pp. 875-877.

3. F. GROS, M. BELJANSKI, M. MACHEBOEUF, « Mode d'action de la pénicilline chez Staphylococcus aureus. Inhibition d'un système enzymatique extrait des bactéries. » C.R. Acad. Sci., 1950, 231, pp. 184-186.

4. F. GROS, M. BELJANSKI, M. MACHEBOEUF, « Action de la pénicilline sur le métabolisme de l'acide ribonucléique chez Staphylococcus aureus. » Bull. Soc. Chim. Biol., 1951, 33, pp.1696-1717.

5. F. GROS, M. BELJANSKI, M. MACHEBOEUF, F. GRUMBACH, F. BOYER, « Activité biologique des combinaisons streptomycine-acides gras . » C.R. Acad., Sci., 1951, 232, pp.764-766.

6. M. BELJANSKI, « Etude de souches bactériennes résistantes à des antibiotiques. Comparaison avec des souches sensibles de mêmes espèces. » Ann. Biol., 1951, 27, pp. 775-780.

7. M. BELJANSKI, « Etude des souches bactériennes résistantes à des antibiotiques. Comparaison avec des souches sensibles de mêmes espèces. » Thèse de Doctorat ès Sciences d'Etat, Université Paris-la Sorbonne, 1951, Paris, Librairie Arnette, 1952.

8. M. BELJANSKI, « Action de la cocarboxylase sur le métabolisme des acides nucléiques chez Staphylococcus aureus sensible et résistant à la streptomycine ». 2ème Congrès Intern. de Biochimie, Paris, 1952. Résumé des communications, 99.

9. M. BELJANSKI, « Comparaison de souches bactériennes résistantes à des antibiotiques avec des souches sensibles de même espèce -I : Cas de la streptomycine. » Ann. Inst. Pasteur, 1952, 83, pp. 80-101.

10. M. BELJANSKI, « Comparaison de souches bactériennes résistantes à des antibiotiques avec des souches sensibles de même espèce - II : Cas de la pénicilline. » Ann. Inst. Pasteur, 1953, 84, pp. 402-408.

11. M. BELJANSKI, « Comparaison de souches bactériennes résistantes à des antibiotiques avec des souches sensibles de même espèce -III : Cas du sulfamide - IV : Cas de l'azoture de sodium. » Ann. Inst. Pasteur, 1953, 84, pp. 756-764.

12. M. BELJANSKI, « Comparaison de souches bactériennes résistantes à la streptomycine avec des souches sensibles de même espèce. » C.R. Acad. Sci., 1953, 236, pp. 1102-1104.

13. M. BELJANSKI, F. GRUMBACH, « Etude biochimique d'une souche de Mycobacterium tuberculosis streptomycino-sensible et d'une souche streptomycino-résistance dérivée de la souche sensible ». C.R. Acad., Sci., 1953, 236, pp. 2111-2113.

14. M. BELJANSKI, « Etude des acides nucléiques de souches bactériennes résistantes à la streptomycine et souches de mêmes espèces mais sensibles à l'antibiotique. » Ann. Inst. Pasteur, 1953, 85, pp. 463-469.

15. M. BELJANSKI, J.GUELFI, « Etude à l'aide du 32P de l'accumulation des acides nucléiques chez Staphylococcus aureus et Salmonella enteritidis résistants et sensibles à la streptomycine. » Ann. Inst. Pasteur, 1954, 86, pp. 115-117.

16. M. BELJANSKI, « L'absence de cytochromes et de certains systèmes enzymatiques dans un nouveau mutant d'Escherichia coli streptomycino-résistant. Comparaison avec la souche sensible dont il dérive ». C.R. Acad., Sci., 1954, 238, pp. 852-854.

17. M. BELJANSKI, « L'action de la ribonucléase et de la désoxyribonucléase sur l'incorporation de glycocolle radioactif dans les protéines de lysats de Micrococcus lysodeikticus. » Biochim. Biophys. Acta. 15, 99. 425-431.

18. M. BELJANSKI, « Isolement de mutants d'Escherichia coli streptomycino-résistants dépourvus d'enzymes respiratoires. Action de l'hémine sur la formation de ces enzymes chez le mutant H-7 ». C.R. Acad., Sci., 1955, 240, pp. 374-376.

19. M. BELJANSKI, « Formation d'enzymes respiratoires chez un mutant d'Escherichia coli streptomycino-résistant ne manifestant pas d'activité respiratoire. » 3ème Congrès Intern. Biochim., Bruxelles, 1955, p. 98 - Résumés des communications. Congres

20. R. LATARJET, M. BELJANSKI, « Photorestoration in porphyrin-less mutants of Escherichia coli. » Microbial Genetic Bulletin, E. Witkin, 1955 - Résumés.

21. M. BELJANSKI, « Reconstitution in vitro de la catalase. » C.R. Acad., Sci., 1955, 241, pp. 1353-1355.

22. R. LATARJET, M. BELJANSKI, « Photorestauration de bactéries dépourvues de porphyrines. » Ann. Inst. Pasteur, 1956, 90, pp. 127-132.

23. M. BELJANSKI, M. S. BELJANSKI, « Sur la formation d'enzymes respiratoires chez un mutant d'Escherichia coli streptomycino-résistant et auxotrophe pour l'hémine. » Ann. Inst. Pasteur, 1957, 92, pp. 396-412.

24. M. BELJANSKI, S. OCHOA, "Protein bio-synthesis by a cell-free bacterial system » Proc. Nat. Acad. Sci. Biochemistry, 1958, 44, pp. 494-500.

25. M. BELJANSKI, M. S. BELJANSKI, VII-ème Congrès Intern. de Microbiol. Stockholm, 1958, Symposium, II. Discussions.

26. M. BELJANSKI, S. OCHOA, "Protein bio-synthesis by a cell-free bacterial system" IV-ème Congrès Intern. Biochim. Vienne, 1958, p. 49 - Résumés des communications.

27. M. BELJANSKI, S. OCHOA, "Protein bio-synthesis by a cell-free bacterial system. II-Further studies on the amino acid incorporation enzyme." Proc. Nat. Acad. Sci., 1958, 44, pp. 1157-1161.

28. M. BELJANSKI, « Identification de quatre kinases spécifiques des diphosphonucléosides dans une préparation enzymatique d'origine bactérienne. » C.R. Acad. Sci., 1959, 248, pp. 1146-1448.

29. M. BELJANSKI, « Synthèse de peptides par un système enzymatique en présence de nucléoside – triphosphates. » C.R. Acad. Sci., 1960, 250, pp. 624-626.

30. M. BELJANSKI, "Protein biosynthesis by a cell-free bacterial system. III-Determination of new peptide bonds; requirements for the 'amino acid incorporation enzyme' in protein biosynthesis" Biochim. Biophys. Acta., 1960, 41, pp. 104-110.

31. M. BELJANSKI, "Protein biosynthesis by a cell-free bacterial system. IV-Exchange of diphosphonucleosides with homologous triphosphonucleosides by the amino acid incorporation enzyme." Biochim. Biophys. Acta., 1960, 41, pp. 111-115.

32. M. BELJANSKI, "Ribonucleoside-5'-triphosphate dependent synthesis of peptides by the purified amino acid incorporation enzyme." Progress in Biophysics and Biophysical Chemistry, Pergamon Press, 1961, 11, p. 238.

33. M. BELJANSKI, « Ribonucléoside-triphosphates et synthèses de peptides spécifiques par des enzymes purifiés. » Bull. Soc. Chim. Biol., 1961,43, pp. 1018-1030.

34. M. BELJANSKI, « Ribonucléoside-triphosphates et synthèse enzymatique de liaisons peptidiques. » Symposium sur les Acides Ribonucléiques et les Polyphosphates." C.N.R.S., 1961, pp. 474-475.

35. M. BELJANSKI, M. S. BELJANSKI, « Synthèses de peptides spécifiques par un système enzymatique purifié d'Alcaligenes faecalis. » Vème Congrès Intern. Biochim. Moscou, 1961, p. 24. Congres

36. M. BELJANSKI, Discussions, Symposium sur la Biosynthèse des Protéines. Vème Congrès Intern. Biochim. Moscou, 1961. Congres

37. J.P. ZALTA, M. BELJANSKI, « Synthèse de peptides par des fractions subcellulaires préparées à partir du foie de rat. » C.R. Acad. Sci. 1961, 253, pp. 567-569

38. M. BELJANSKI, M. S. BELJANSKI, T. LOVINY, « Rôle des polypeptide-synthétases dans la formation de peptides spécifiques en présence de ribonucléoside-triphosphates. » Biochim. Biophys. Acta., 1962, 56, pp. 559-570.

39. M. BELJANSKI, "Participation of an RNA fraction in peptide synthesis in the presence of a purified enzyme system from Alcaligenes faecalis." Biochim. Biophys. Res. Comm., 1962, 8, pp. 15-19.

40. M. BELJANSKI, M. S. BELJANSKI, « Acide aminé - acide ribonucléique , intermédiaire dans la synthèse des liasons peptidiques. » VI- Biochim. Biophys. Acta., 1963, 72, pp. 585-597.

41. M. BELJANSKI, « ARN-messager: intermédiaire direct dans la synthèse des liaisons peptidiques. » Colloque International du C.N.R.S., Marseille, 1963, pp. 39-44. (Mécanismes de régulation des activités cellulaires chez les micro-organismes).

42. M. BELJANSKI, C. FISHER, M. S. BELJANSKI, « Le RNA messager, accepteur spécifique des L-acides aminés en présence d'enzymes bactériennes. » C.R. Acad. Sci., 1963,257, pp. 547-549.

43. M. BELJANSKI, C. FISHER, « Les ARN messagers gouvernant la synthèse « in vitro » des chaînes peptidiques en présence de polypeptides synthétases. » Pathologie-Biologie, 1965,13, pp. 198-203.

44. M. BELJANSKI, "Messenger RNA dependent Synthesis of peptides by purified bacterial enzymes." Bioch-Zeits, 1965, 342, pp. 392-399.

45. M. BELJANSKI, « L'ARN isolé du virus de la mosaïque jaune du Navet, accepteur des l-acides aminés en présence d'enzymes bactériennes. » Bull. Soc. Chim. Biol. 1965, 47, pp. 1645-1652.

46. M. BELJANSKI, N. VAPAILLE, « Rôle des triterpènes dans l'attachement des l-acides aminés par des « ARN matriciels. » Eur. J. of Clin. Biol. Res., 1971, pp. 897-908.

47. M. BELJANSKI, P. BOURGAREL, « Isolement de di- et trinucléotides, sites spécifiques d'attachement d'arginine et de valine dans des ARN d' origines différentes ». C.R. Acad. Sci., 1967, 264, pp. 1760-1763 (série D).

48. M. BELJANSKI, C. FISCHER-FERRARO, « Nouvelle méthode de purification des polypeptides synthétases. » C.R. Acad. Sci., 1967, 264, pp. 411-414 (série D).

49. M. BELJANSKI, C. FISCHER-FERRARO, P. BOURGAREL, « Identification des sites d'attachement spécifiques d'arginine et de valine dans des ARN d'origines différentes. » VIII- European J. Biochem., 1968, 4, pp. 184-189.

50. C. FISCHER-FERRARO, M. BELJANSKI, « Nouvelle méthode de purification des polypeptides synthétases. » VII- European J. Biochem., 1968, 4, pp. 118-125.

51. M. BELJANSKI, P. BOURGAREL, « Isolement et caractérisation d'un RNA matriciel d'Alcaligenes faecalis. » C.R. Acad. Sci., 1968, 266, pp. 845-847.

52. M. BELJANSKI, M.S. BELJANSKI, « Synthèse chez Escherichia coli des ARN dont la structure primaire diffère de celle de l'ADN. » C.R. Acad. Sci., 1968, 267, pp. 1058-1060 (série D).

53. M. BELJANSKI, M.S. BELJANSKI, P. BOURGAREL, J. CHASSAGNE, « Synthèse chez les bactéries d'ARN nouveaux n'étant pas la copie de l'ADN. » C.R. Acad. Sci., 1969, 269, pp. 240-243 (série D).

54. M. BELJANSKI, P. BOURGAREL, M.S. BELJANSKI, « Showdomycine et biosynthèse d'ARN non complémentaire de l'ADN » - I -. Ann. Inst. Pasteur, 1970, 118, pp. 253-276.

55. M. BELJANSKI, P. BOURGAREL, M.S. BELJANSKI, "Drastic alteration of ribosomal RNA and ribosomal proteins in showdomycin-resistant Escherichia coli." Proc. Nat. Aca. Sci. (USA), 1971,68, pp. 491-495.

56. M. PLAWECKI, M. BELJANSKI, « Transcription par la polynucléotide phosphorylase de l'ARN associé à l'ADN d'Escherichia coli. » C.R. Acad. Sci., 1971, 273, pp. 827-830 (série D).

57. M. BELJANSKI, M.S. BELJANSKI, P. BOURGAREL, « ARN transformants porteurs de caractères héréditaires chez Escherichia coli showdomycino-résistant. » C.R. Acad. Sci., 1971, 272, pp. 2107-2110 (série D).

58. M. BELJANSKI, M.S. BELJANSKI, P. BOURGAREL, « « Episome à ARN » porté par l'ADN d'Escherichia coli sauvage et showdomycino-résistant. » C.R. Acad. Sci., 1971, 272, pp. 2736-3739 (série D).

59. M. BELJANSKI, M.S. BELJANSKI, P. MANIGAULT, P. BOURGAREL, "Transformation of Agrobacterium tumefaciens into a non-oncogenic species by an Escheria coli RNA" Proc. Nat. Aca. Sci. (USA), 1972, 69, pp. 191-195.

60. M. BELJANSKI, « Synthèse in vitro de l'ADN sur une matrice d'ARN par une transcriptase d'Escherichia coli. » C.R. Acad. Sci., 1972, 274, pp.2801-2804 (série D).

61. M. BELJANSKI, C. BONISSOL, P. KONA, "Transformation des cellules K.B. induites par la showdomycine." C.R. Acad. Sci., 1972,274, pp. 3116-3119 (série D).

62. M. BELJANSKI, P. MANIGAULT, "Genetic transformation of bacteria by RNA and loss of oncogenic power properties of Agrobacterium tumefaciens. Transforming RNA as template for DNA synthesis." Sixth Miles International Symposium on Molecular Biology. Ed. F. Beers and R.C. Tilghman. The John Hopkins University Press, Baltimore, 1972, pp. 81-97.

63. M. BELJANSKI, « Séparation de la transcriptase inverse de l'ADN polymérase ADN dépendante. Analyse de l'ADN synthétisé sur le modèle de l'ARN transformant. » C.R. Acad. Sci., 1973, 276, pp. 1625-1628 (série D).

64. M. BELJANSKI, M. PLAWECKI, "Transforming RNA as a template directing RNA and DNA synthesis in bacteria." In Niu and Segal (eds), The Role of RNA in Reproduction and Development. North Holland Publ.Co., 1973, pp. 203-224.

65. M. PLAWECKI, M. BELJANSKI, « Synthèse in vitro d'un ARN utilisé comme amorceur pour la réplication de l'ADN. » C.R. Acad. Sci., 1974, 278, pp. 1413-1416 (série D).

66. M. BELJANSKI, Y. AARON-DA-CUNHA, M.S. BELJANSKI, P. MANIGAULT, P. BOURGAREL, "Isolation of the tumor-inducing RNA from Oncogenic and Nononcogenic Agrobacterium tumefaciens." Proc. Nat. Acad. Sci. (USA), 1974,71, pp. 1585-1589.

67. M. BELJANSKI, M.S. BELJANSKI, « RNA-bound Reverse Transcriptase in Escherichia coli and in vitro synthesis of a complementary DNA ». Biochemical genetics, 1974, 12, pp. 163-180.

68. M. BELJANSKI, P. MANIGAULT, M.S. BELJANSKI, Y. AARON-DA-CUNHA, "Genetic transformation of Agrobacterium B_6 tumefaciens by RNA and nature of the tumor inducing principle." First Intern. Congress of the Intern. Assoc. of Microbiol. Soc. Tokyo I.A.M.S., 1974,1, pp.132-141.

69. M. BELJANSKI, M. S. BELJANSKI, M. PLAWECKI, P. MANIGAULT, « ARN-fragments, amorceurs nécessaires à la réplication « in vitro » des ADN. » C.R. Acad. Sci., 1975,280, pp. 363-366 (série D).

70. M. BELJANSKI, L. CHAUMONT, C. BONISSOL, M. S. BELJANSKI, « ARN-fragments inhibiteurs « in vivo » de la multiplication des virus du fibrome de Shope et de la vaccine. » C.R. Acad. Sci., 1975, 280, pp. 783-786 (série D).

71. M. BELJANSKI, « ARN-amorceurs riches en nucléotides G et A indispensables à la réplication in vitro de l'ADN des phages YX174 et lambda. » C.R. Acad. Sci., 1975, 280, pp. 783-786 (série D).

72. L. LE GOFF, Y. AARON-DA-CUNHA, M. BELJANSKI, "RNA fraction from several nononcogenic strains of Agrobacterium tumefaciens as tumor inducing agent in Datura stramonium." XIIth Intern. Bot. Congress. Résumés. Leningrad, 1975. Congres

73. M. BELJANSKI, Y. AARON-DA-CUNHA, "RNA fraction from others sources than Agrobacterium tumefaciens as tumor inducing agent in Datura stramonium." Workshop Third Intern. Congress of Virology, Madrid, 1975, p. 15.

74. L. LE GOFF, Y. AARON-DA-CUNHA, M. BELJANSKI, « Un ARN extrait d'Agrobacterium tumefaciens souches oncogènes et non oncogènes, éléments indispensables à l'induction des tumeurs chez Datura stramonium. » Canadian J. of Microbiology, 1976, 22, pp. 694-701.

75. M. BELJANSKI, Y. AARON-DA-CUNHA, "Particular small size RNA and RNA fragments from different origins as tumor inducing agents in in Datura stramoium." Molec. Biol. Reports, 1976, 2, pp. 497-506.

76. S.K. DUTTA, M. BELJANSKI, P. BOURGAREL, "Endogenous RNA-bound RNA dependent DNA polymerase activity in Neurospora crassa." Exp. Mycology, 1977, 1, pp. 173-182.

77. L. LE GOFF, Y. AARON-DA-CUNHA, M. BELJANSKI, « Polyribonucleotides, agents inducteurs et inhibiteurs des tissus tumoraux. » Conf. Intern. Montpellier (1978) - Résumés.

78. M. BELJANSKI, P. BOURGAREL, M.S. BELJANSKI, « Découpage des ARN ribosomiques d'Escherichia coli par la ribonucléase U2 et transcription in vitro des ARN-fragments en ADN complémentaires. » C.R. Acad. Sci., 1978, 286, pp. 1825-1828 (série D).

79. M. BELJANSKI, M. PLAWECKI, P. BOURGAREL, M. S. BELJANSKI, « Nouvelles substances (R.L.B.) actives dans la leucopoïèse et la formation des plaquettes. » Bull. Acad. Nat. Med., 1978, 162, Volume n°6, pp. 475-781.

80. M. STROUN, Ph. ANKER, M. BELJANSKI, J. HENRI, Ch. LEDERREY, M. OJHA, P. MAURICE, "Presence of RNA in the nucleo-protein complex spontaneously released by human lymphocytes and frog auricles." Cancer Res., 1978, 38, pp. 3546-3551.

81. M. BELJANSKI, L. LE GOFF, Y. AARON-DA-CUNHA, "Special short dual-action RNA fragments can both induce and inhibit crown-gall tumors." Proc. 4th Conf. Plant Path. Bacteria Angers, 1978, pp. 207-220.

82. M. BELJANSKI, L. LE GOFF, « Stimulation de l'induction - ou inhibition du développement - des tumeurs de crown-gall par des ARN-fragments U2. Interférence de l'auxine. » C.R. Acad. Sci., 1979, 288, pp. 147-150 (série D).

83. M. BELJANSKI, M. PLAWECKI, "Particular RNA fragments as promoters of leucocytes and platelets formations in rabbits." Exp. Cell Biol., 1979, 47, pp. 218-225.

84. M. BELJANSKI, "Oncotest: a DNA assay system for the screening of carcinogenic substances." IRCS Medical science, 1979, 47, pp. 218-225.

85. L. LE GOFF, M. BELJANSKI, "Cancer/anti-cancer dual action drugs in crown-gall tumors." IRCS Medical Science, 1979,7, p. 476.

86. M. BELJANSKI, "Oligoribo-nucleotides, promoters of leucocyte and platelet genesis in animals depleted by anticancer drugs." NCI-EORTC Symposium on nature, prevention and treatment of clinical toxicity of anticancer agents. Institut Bordet, Bruxelles, 1980. Congres

87. M. BELJANSKI, M. PLAWECKI, P. BOURGAREL, M.S. BELJANSKI, "Short chain RNA fragments as promoters of leucocyte and platelet genesis in animals depleted by anti-cancer drugs." In the Role of RNA in Development and Reproduction. Sec. Int. Symposium, April 25-30, 1980, pp. 79-113. Science Press Beijing. M.C. Niu and H.H. Chuang Eds Van Nostrand Reinhold Company.

88. M. BELJANSKI, P. BOURGAREL, M.S. BELJANSKI, "Correlation between in vitro DNA synthesis, DNA strand separation and in vivo multiplication of cancer cells." Expl. Cell. Biol., 49,1981, pp.220-231.

89. M. PLAWECKI, M. BELJANSKI, "Comparative study of Escherichia coli, endotoxin, hydrocortisone and Beljanski Leucocyte Restorers activity in cyclophosphamide-treated rabbits." Proc. of the Soc. for Exp. Biol. and Med., 168, 1981, pp.408-413.

90. M. BELJANSKI, L. LE GOFF, M.S. BELJANSKI, "Differential susceptibility of cancer and normal DNA templates allows the detection of carcinogens and anticancer drugs." Third NCI-EORTS Symp. on new drugs in Cancer Therapy, Institut Bordet, Bruxelles, 1981.

91. L. LE GOFF, M. BELJANSKI, "Crown-gall tumor stimulation or inhibition: correlation with DNA strand separation." Proc. Fifth Conf. Plant Path. Bact. Cali, 1981, p. 295-307.

92. M. BELJANSKI, M.S. BELJANSKI, "Selective inhibition of in vitro synthesis of cancer DNA by alkaloids of b-carboline class." Expl. Cell. Biol., 50, 1982, pp.79-87.

93. L. LE GOFF, M. BELJANSKI, "Agonist and/or antagonists effects of plant hormones and an anticancer alkaloid on plant DNA structure and activity" IRCS Med. Sci., 10, 1982, pp. 689-690.

94. M. BELJANSKI, L. LE GOFF, A. FAIVRE-AMIOT, "Preventive and curative anticancer drug. Application to Crown-gall tumors." Acta Horticulturae, n°125, 1982, pp. 239-248.

95. M. BELJANSKI, « Oncotest: dépistage des potentiels cancérogènes et spécifiquement anti-cancéreux. Conceptions et perspectives nouvelles en cancérologie. » Environnement et nouvelle médecine. n°2, 1982, pp.18-23.

96. M. BELJANSKI, L. LE GOFF, M. S. BELJANSKI, "In vitro Screening of Carcinogens using DNA of the His-Mutant of Salmonella typhimurium." Expl. Cell. Biol., 50, 1982, pp. 271-280.

97. M. BELJANSKI, L. LE GOFF, "Tumor promoter (TPA), DNA chain opening and unscheduled DNA synthesis." IRCS Med. Sci., 11, 1983, pp. 363-364.

98. M. BELJANSKI, M. PLAWECKI, P. BOURGAREL, M.S. BELJANSKI, "Leukocyte recovery with short-chain RNA fragments in cyclophosphamide-treated rabbits." Cancer Treatment Reports, 67, 1983, pp. 611-619.

99. M. BELJANSKI, "The Regulation of DNA Replication and Transcription. The Role of Trigger Molecules in Normal and Malignant Gene Expression." Experimental Biology and Medicine, vol. 8, Karger (1983), pp. 1-190.

100. M. BELJANSKI, M.S. BELJANSKI, "Three alkaloids as selective destroyers of the proliferative capacity of cancer cells." IRCS Med. Sci., 12, 1984, pp. 587-588.

101. L. LE GOFF, J. ROUSSAUX, Y. AARON-DA-CUNHA, M. BELJANSKI, "Growth inhibition of crown-gall tissues in relation to the structure and activity of DNA." Physiol. Plant., 64, 1985, pp 177-184.

102. L. LE GOFF, M. BELJANSKI, "The in vitro effects of opines and other compounds on DNAs originating from bacteria and from healthy and tumorous plant tissues." Expl. Cell. Biol., 53, 1985, pp. 335-350.

103. M. BELJANSKI, « Activation et inactivation des gènes: Incidence en cancérologie ». Aspect de la recherche. Université Paris-Sud, 1985, pp. 56-62

104. M. BELJANSKI, M.S. BELJANSKI, "Three alkaloids as selective destroyers of cancer cells in mice. Synergy with classic anticancer drugs." Oncology, 43, 1986, pp 198-203.

105. M. BELJANSKI, L. LE GOFF, "Analysis of small RNA species: phylogenetic trends." In DNA Systematics, vol.I: Evolution. Ed. S.K. Dutta CRC Press, Inc. Florida (1986), pp.81-105.

106. M. BELJANSKI, T. NAWROCKI, L. LE GOFF, "Possible role of markers synthesized during cancer evolution: I- Markers in mamalian tissues." IRCS Med. Sci. 14, 1986, pp. 809-810.

107. L. LE GOFF, M. BELJANSKI, "Possible role of markers synthesized during cancer evolution: II- Markers in crown-gall tissues." IRCS Med. Sci. 14, 1986, pp. 811-812.

108. M. BELJANSKI, L. LE GOFF, M.S. BELJANSKI, « Régulation des gènes, cancer et prevention. » Médecines nouvelles, 15, 1986, pp. 57-86.

109. M. BELJANSKI, "Terminal deoxynucleotidyl transferase and ribonuclease activities in purified hepatitis-B antigen." Med. Sci. Res., 15, 1987, pp. 529-530.

110. M. BELJANSKI, S.K. DUTTA, "Differential synthesis and replication of DNA in the Neurospora crassa slime mutant versus normal cells: Role of carcinogens." Oncology, 44, 1987, pp. 327-330.

111. S.K. DUTTA, M. BELJANSKI, "Particular RNA primer from growth medium differentially stimulates in vitro DNA synthesis and in vivo cell

growth of Neurospora crassa and its slime mutant." Current Genetics, 12, 1987, pp. 283-289.

112. M. BELJANSKI, L.C. NIU, M.S. BELJANSKI, S. YAN, M.C. NIU, "Iron stimulated RNA-dependent DNA polymerase Activity from goldfish eggs." Cellular and Molecular Biology, 34, 1988, pp. 17-25.

113. L. LE GOFF, M. WICKER, M. BELJANSKI, "Reversible biophysical changes of DNAs from in vitro cultured non-tumour cells." Med. Sci. Res., 16, 1988, pp. 359-360.

114. M. STROUN, P. ANKER, P. MAURICE, J. LYAUTEY, C. LEDERREY, M. BELJANSKI, "Neoplastic Characteristics of the DNA Found in the Plasma of Cancer Patients." Oncology, 16, 1989, pp. 318-322.

115. M. BELJANSKI, M.S. BELJANSKI, M. GRANDI "Resultati preliminari dell'impiego di tre alcaloidi nel carcinoma prostatico." In Tumori, Instituo Nationale per le studio ed la cura dei tumori (ed. Lambrosiana), Vol. 75, suppl. 4, 1989.

116. M. BELJANSKI, "Cancer therapy: A New Approach." Deutsche Zeitschrift für Onkologie 5, 22, 1990, pp. 145-152.

117. M. BELJANSKI, « Cancer et Sida. Nouvelles approches thérapeutiques. » 5èmes Entretiens Internationaux de Monaco, 21-24 novembre 1990 (Ed. du Rocher), pp. 25-34.

118. D. DONADIO, R. LORHO, J.E. CAUSSE, T. NAWROCKI, M. BELJANSKI, "RNA fragments (RLB) and Tolerance of Cytostatic Treatments in Hematology: A Preliminary Study about Two Non-Hodgkin Malignant Lymphoma Cases." Deutsche Zeitschrift für Onkologie, 23, 2, 1991, pp. 33-35.

119. M. BELJANSKI, "Reverse Transcriptases in Bacteria: Small RNAs as Genetic Vectors and Biological Modulators." Brazil. J. Genetics, 14, 4, 1991, pp. 873-896.

120. M. BELJANSKI, "Radioprotection of Irradiated Mice - Mechanisms and Synergistic Action of WR-2721 and R.L.B." Deutsche Zeitschrift für Onkologie, 23, 6, 1991, pp. 155-159.

121. M. BELJANSKI, "Overview: BLRs as Inducers of *in vivo* Leucocyte and Platelet Genesis." Deutsche Zeitschrift für Onkologie, 24, 2, 1992, pp. 45-45.

122. M. BELJANSKI, "A New Approach to Cancer Therapy." Proceedings of the international seminar: Traditional Medicine: A Challenge of the 21st Century, 7-9 Nov. 1992, Calcutta (Ed. in chief Biswapati Mukherjee).

123. M. BELJANSKI, S. CROCHET, M.S. BELJANSKI, "PB100: A Potent and Selective Inhibitor of Human BCNU Resistant Glioblastoma Cell Multiplication." Anticancer Research, vol. 13, n°6A, Nov. Dec. 1993, pp. 2301-2308.

124. M. BELJANSKI, S. CROCHET, "Differential effects of ferritin, calcium, zinc and gallic acid on *in vitro* proliferation of human glioblastoma cells and normal astrocytes." J. Lab. Clin. Med. 123:547-555, 1994.

125. M. BELJANSKI, S. CROCHET, "The selective anticancer agent PB-100 inhibits interleukin-6 induced enhancement of glioblastoma cell proliferation in vitro." International Journal of Oncology, 5:873-879, 1994.

126. M. BELJANSKI, S. CROCHET, "Selective inhibitor (PB-100) of human glioblastoma cell multiplication." Journal of Neuro-Oncology, Vol. 21, N°1, p. 62, 1994.

127. J.E. CAUSSE, T. NAWROCKI, M. BELJANSKI, "Human Skin Fibrosis Rnase Search for a Biological Inhibitor-Regulator." Deutsche Zeitschrift für Onkologie, 26, 5, 1994, pp. 137-139.

128. M. BELJANSKI, S. CROCHET, "The anticancer agent PB100 concentrates in the nucleus and nucleoli of human glioblastoma cells but does not enter normal astrocytes." International Journal of Oncology 7:81-85, 1995.

129. M. BELJANSKI, "Novel selective nontoxic anticancer and antiviral agents." International Journal of Oncology Vol. 7. supplement, p. 983, October 1995.

130. M. BELJANSKI, S. CROCHET, "The selective anticancer agents PB-100 and BG-8 are active against human melanoma cells, but do not affect non malignant fibroblasts." International Journal of Oncology 8:1143-1148,1996.

131. M. BELJANSKI, S. CROCHET, "Mitogenic effect of several interleukins, neuromediators and hormones on human glioblastoma cells, and its inhibition by the selective anticancer agent PB-100." Deutsche Zeitschrift für Onkologie, 28, 1, 1996, pp.14-2.

132. M. BELJANSKI, "De novo synthesis of DNA - like molecules by polyaudeotide phosphorylase in vitro." J. Mol. Evol. 1996, 42:493-499.

133. M. BELJANSKI, "The anticancer agent PB-100, selectively active on malignant cells, inhibits multiplication of sixteen malignant cell lines, even multidrug resistant." Genetics and Molecular Biology, 23, 1, 29-33 (2000)

Appendix 2: *Pao pereira* content comparison chart (Flavopereirine)

The Beljanski Foundation procured nine samples of dietary supplements from the United States and Europe for comparison. The objective was to compare the levels of flavopereirine to see if the beneficial compound in the products were similar in content across several brands.

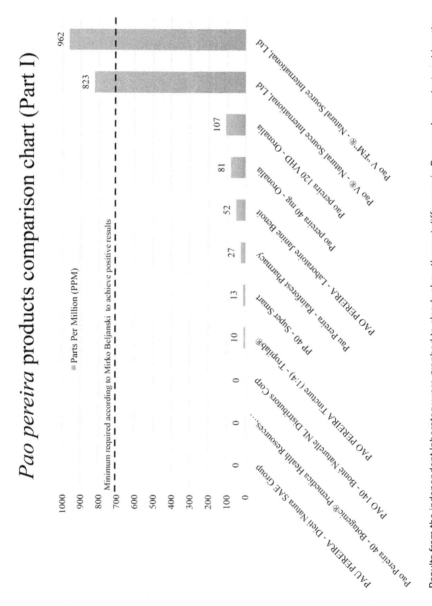

Results from the independent laboratory were graphed to clearly show the vast difference in *Pao pereira* products sold on the market. (© The Beljanski Foundation, Inc.)

Pao pereira products comparison chart (Part II)

	Parts Per Million (PPM)
PAU PEREIRA - Dieti Natura SAE Group - Lot P160 300B (Switzerland)	0
Pao Pereira 40 - Botagenic® Premedica Health Resources, LLC. - Lot 1607121 (U.S.)	0
PAO 140 - Bonté Naturelle NL Distributors Corp - No lot number (Canada)	0
PAO PEREIRA Tincture (1:4) - Tropilab® - No lot number (U.S.)	10
PP 40 - Super Smart - Lot 16055A (Luxembourg)	13
Pau Pereira - Rainforest Pharmacy - Lot RPx 081114 (U.S.)	27
PAO PEREIRA - Laboratoire Janine Benoit - Lot PAO 916 (Spain)	52
Pao pereira 40 mg - Oronalia - Lot 088.1.170125 (Luxembourg)	81
Pao pereira 120 VHD - Oronalia - Lot 088.3.170120 (Luxembourg)	107
Pao V® - Natural Source International, Ltd. - Lot 1-840 V-1607 (U.S.)	823
Pao V FM® - Natural Source International, Ltd. - Lot 2-528-1701 (U.S.)	962

The Beljanski Foundation's research on *Pao pereira* was done with samples provided by Natural Source International. The quality of those samples has led to the following publications:

Pancreatic cancer

Yu, Jun, Jeanne Drisko, and Qi Chen. "Inhibition of Pancreatic Cancer and Potentiation of Gemcitabine Effects by the Extract of *Pao pereira*." *Oncology Reports* 30, no. 1 (July 2013): 149-56.

Ovarian cancer

Yu, Jun, and Qi Chen. "The Plant Extract of *Pao pereira* Potentiates Carboplatin Effects Against Ovarian Cancer." *Pharmaceutical Biology* 52, no. 1 (January 2014): 36-43.

Prostate cancer

Bemis, Debra L., Jillian L. Capodice, Manisha Desai, Aaron E. Katz, and Ralph Buttyan. "β-Carboline Alkaloid-Enriched Extract from the Amazonian Rain Forest Tree *Pao pereira* Suppresses Prostate Cancer Cells." *Journal of the Society for Integrative Oncology* 7, no. 2 (Spring 2009): 59-65.

Chang, Cunjie, Wei Zhao, Bingxian Xie, Yongming Deng, Tao Han, Yangyan Cui, Yundong Dai, Zhen Zhang, Jimin Gao, Hongqian Guo, and Jun Yan. "*Pao pereira* Extract Suppresses Castration-Resistant Prostate Cancer Cell Growth, Survival, and Invasion Through Inhibition of NFκB Signaling." *Integrative Cancer Therapies* 13, no. 3 (May 2014): 249-58.

Appendix 3: **RNA Fragments Comparison Chart**

Comparison between
E.coli RNA and yeast RNA

Beljanski Method E.coli RNA Fragments   **Yeast-based RNA Fragments**

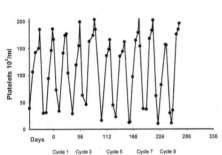 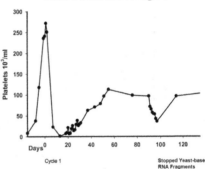

Figure 1 Breast Cancer Patient with Metastatic Disease to Flat Bones with Two Prior Chemotherapy Regimens—Current Regimen is Doxorubicin.

Figure 2 Metastatic Lung Cancer Patient (Long Bones/Lymph Nodes) Failed Three Prior Regimens and Undergoing Ifosamide/Doxorubicin/Decabazine.

Comparaison between E.coli RNA and yeast RNA Source: Levin, Robert D., Maryann Daehler, James F. Grutsch, John L. Hall, Digant Gupta, and Christopher G. Lis. "Dose Escalation Study of an Anti-Thrombocytopenic Agent in Patients with Chemotherapy Induced Thrombocytopenia." *BMC Cancer 10,* no. 565 (October 19, 2010).

Appendix 4: **Retrocitiation by HOWARD M. TEMIN**

RETROCITATION

SIR–In my News and Views article «Reverse Transcriptases. Retrons in Bacteria» (ref.[1]) I stated «no such reverse transcriptase seemed to exist in bacteria». M. Beljanski has since called my attention to his publications on reverse transcriptase in bacteria[2-5]. This work was confirmed in several Soviet publications[6-9]. It will be of interest to see if these activities are related to retrons.

HOWARD M. TEMIN

McArdle Laboratory,
University of Wisconsin,
Madison, Wisconsin 53706, USA

1. Temin, H.M. *Nature* 339, 254-255 (1989).
2. Beljanski, M. *C. r. hebd. Séanc. Acad. Sci., Paris* D274, 2801-2804 (1972).
3. Beljanski, M. *C. r. hebd. Séanc. Acad. Sci., Paris* D276, 1625-1628 (1973).
4. Beljanski, M. & Beljanski M., *Biochem. Genet.* 17, 163-180 (1974).
5. Beljanski, M., Bourgarel, P. & Beljanski M.S. *C. r. hebd. Séanc. Acad. Sci., Paris* D286, 1825-1828 (1978).
6. Romashchenko, A.G. *et al. Dokl. Akad. Nauk SSSR* 233, 734-737 (1977).
7. Lushnikova, T.P. *et al. Molec. Biol.* 12, 1163-1171 (1978).
8. Vorob'eva, N.V. *et al. Molec. Biol.* 16, 977-983 (1982).
9. Grabkina, O.A., *et al. Molec. Biol.* 17, 830-838 (1988).

NATURE - VOL 342 - 7 DECEMBER 1989

Appendix 5: **Letter from Dr. Sten Friberg**

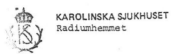

KAROLINSKA SJUKHUSET
Radiumhemmet

80 11 03

Dr. M. Beljanski
Laboratoire de Pharmacodynamie
Université de Paris-Sud
Faculté des Sciences
Pharmaceutiques & Biologiques
rue Jean-Baptiste-Clement
F-92290 Chatenay-Malabry
FRANCE

Dear Dr Beljanski,

At the E.O.R.T.C. meeting in Brussels in September
this year, you gave a very interesting paper entilted:
"Oligoribonucleotides ..... "

I wonder if you could take the trouble to send me
copies of all papers and manuscripts dealing with
those studies. Your ideas and results are simply
fascinating.

Thanking you in advance

Yours sincerely

Sten Friberg, M.D., Ph.D.
Dept. General Oncology
Radiumhemmet
Karolinska Hospital
104 01 STOCKHOLM
Sweden

ACKNOWLEDGMENTS

would like to express my gratitude to the teams of CIRIS, The Beljanski Foundation, and Natural Source International, Ltd. Without you, I wouldn't have a story to tell. And a very special thanks to the Weidlich family for the friendship and loyalty they have demonstrated to my family over the past thirty years.

To Dr. Michael Schachter, for all his positive influence at every turn of this adventure.

I am especially grateful to Alex Lubarsky, who was the first person to tell me that I could and should write a book.

Merci beaucoup to my mother, Monique Beljanski, who offered me, beyond her loving presence and support, her valuable memories, as well as her always wise comments.

To Bob Armstrong and Jacob Jaskiewicz for their sound professional advice. To Loraine Degraff and Patricia Ross for their precious editing.

To Anne Akers, who saw me through the first draft and helped to get this book published.

To David Hancock and the entire team at Morgan James for their wonderful support along the complicated publishing process and special thanks to Aubrey Kosa for her kindness and patience.

To Oriela Cuevas for bringing her organizational skills and helping to get the word out.

To Glenn Zagoren for his friendship, enthusiasm, and brilliant ideas.

Last but not least: To the many people who provided support when I was overwhelmed with the writing process and who talked things over, read, wrote, offered comments, allowed me to quote their remarks and assisted in the editing, proofreading and design.

I beg forgiveness of all those who have been with me over the course of the years and whose names I have failed to mention.

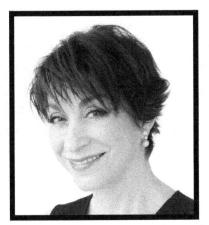

Sylvie Beljanski (Photograph: Ron Contarsy)

ABOUT THE AUTHOR

Sylvie Beljanski was born in New York City after her father, Mirko Beljanski, Ph.D. came to New York to pursue a two-year fellowship with Nobel Prize winner, Severo Ochoa, known for his DNA research on living cells. Raised and educated in Paris, she completed her undergraduate studies at The Sorbonne. After receiving her law degree, she was admitted to the French Bar.

In 1996, Ms. Beljanski founded Natural Source International, Ltd., a company that brings together science and nature to create innovative natural/organic health and beauty products. These well-known products are now used around the world.

In 1999, Ms. Beljanski founded The Beljanski Foundation, a registered non-profit, whose mission is to further Dr. Beljanski's research within a network of high-profile research institutions. Since then, she has been serving as Vice President of the Foundation, relentlessly spreading the word and educating the public about the effects of environmental toxins on our health.

Ms. Beljanski is a sought-after speaker at health and wellness conferences globally, where she has educated thousands of people about the importance of detoxification as a defense against harmful toxins that can cause serious disease and infections. She recommends The Beljanski Approach to Wellness as a practical means to avoid environmental toxins, remove them, and repair the cellular process.

In 2018, Ms. Beljanski will be opening the doors to Maison Beljanski, a new building in the heart of Manhattan, and dedicated to the legacy of her father, Dr. Beljanski. The first floor, home of The Beljanski Foundation, will also serve as a site for hosting numerous conferences on different aspects of health and wellness.

Ms. Beljanski has previously produced two movies and authored one book.

Movies:

- *The Beljanski Legacy* | 22-minute documentary in both French and in English | Available on Youtube

- *Politiquement Incorrecte, mais Scientifiquement Exacte, L'Histoire Beljanski: des Molécules et des Hommes*© | 53-minute documentary in French | Available on Youtube

Other book:

- *Beljanski: Cancer, Santé et Prévention* | Editions Guy Trédaniel ISBN: 978-2-8132-0849-1

Beljanski has been featured by select media, including articles with USA TODAY, Marie Claire, Townsend Letter, The American Chiropractor, Men's Health, The Doctor's Prescription for Healthy Living. She was also interviewed on NBC News TV Channel 4 in New York City.

A sample of her recent conference presentations includes:

- Navel Expo NYC
- Navel Expo Long Island
- New Life Expo

- Annie Appleseed Project
- European Council of Integrative Medicine
- MEDNAT Expo (Switzerland)
- Integrative Healthcare Symposium
- Primevère Exhibition at EUREXPO (France)
- ADNO: Association for the Development of Orthomolecular Nutrition (France)

She is an active member of: National Association of Professional Women; French-American Chamber of Commerce; Greater New York Chamber of Commerce; The Fashion Group International; and The Luxury Marketing Council.

She resides in New York City. Her blog can be found at: www.thebeljanskiblog.com.

RESOURCES

The Beljanski Foundation, Inc.
Email: info@beljanski.org
Website: www.beljanski.org
Tel: 646 808 5583 (Monday to Friday 9am to 6pm EST)

Association CIRIS
BP9
17550 Dolus-d'Oléron
FRANCE
Website: wwww.beljanski.info
Tel: +33 474 56 58 00

Natural Source International, Ltd.
Email: info@natural-source.com
Website: www.natural-source.com
Tel: 212 308 7066 (Monday to Friday 9am to 6pm EST)

Maison Beljanski
317 East 53rd Street,
New York, NY 10022
Email: info@maisonbeljanski.com
Website: www.maisonbeljanski.com

Health Media Group, Inc.
Post Office Box 40
Cedarhurst, NY 11516
Email: info@healthmedia.us
Website: www.navelexpo.com
Tel: 516 596 8974

Alliance for Natural Health
3525 Piedmont rd. Ne, Bld. 6 ste. 310,
Atlanta, GA 30305
Website: www.anh-usa.org
Tel: 800 230 2762

Annie Appleseed Project
7319 Serrano Terrace,
Delray Beach, FL 33446-2215
Email: annieappleseedpr@aol.com
Website: www.annieappleseedproject.org
Tel: 561 749 0084

HSI Members Alert
Post Office Box 913
Frederick, MD 21705-0913
Website: www.hsionline.com

Best Answer For Cancer Foundation
8127 mesa, b-206, #243
Austin, TX 78759
Email: admin@bestanswerforcancer.org
Website: www.bestanswerforcancer.org
Tel: 512 342 8181

The Schachter Center For Complementary Medicine
2 Executive Blvd, Suite 202,
Suffern, NY 10901
Email: office@mbschachter.com
Website: www.mbschachter.com
Tel: 845 368 4700

Jillian Capodice, LAC
Department of urology, Mount Sinai Health System
625 Madison Avenue 2nd floor, Mount Sinai Health System,
New York, NY 10022
Website: www.mountsinai.org/profiles/jillian-l-capodice
Tel: 646 629-0244

R.G.C.C. USA LLC
Branch office in the USA, North America continent & Canada
3105 Main Street,
Rowlett, TX 75088
Website: www.rgccusa.com
Tel: 214 299 9449

Books
The Secret to Long Life in Your DNA: The Beljanski Approach to Cellular Health
Hervé Janecek. ISBN 1594772592

Cancer's Cause, Cancer's Cure: The Truth about Cancer, Its Causes, Cures, and Prevention.
Dr. Morton Walker. ISBN 1936449102

Extraordinary Healing: How the Discoveries of Mirko Beljanski, the World's First Green Molecular Biologist, Can Protect and Restore Your Health
L. Stephen Coles. ISBN 189391089X

Natural Cancer Cures: The Definitive Guide to Using Dietary Supplements to Fight and Prevent Cancer
The Doctors' Prescription for Healthy Living Magazine. ISBN 1893910520

Beljanski: Cancer, Santé et Prévention
Monique Beljanski and Sylvie Beljanski. ISBN: 978-2-8132-0849-1

Cancer, les huit erreurs à éviter pour optimiser votre traitement et multiplier vos chances
Jean-Paul Le Perlier. ISBN 978-2-8132-1430-0

Beljanski et la cancérogénèse
Monique Beljanski. ISBN 978-2-36071-022-5

Mirko Beljanski ou la chronique d'une "fatwa" scientifique
Monique Beljanski. ISBN 0-9671304-1-7

Movies
The Beljanski Legacy
22-minute documentary in both French and in English. Available on YouTube

Politiquement Incorrecte, mais Scientifiquement Exacte, L'Histoire Beljanski : des Molécules et des Hommes©
53-minute documentary in French. Available on YouTube

Articles
"Integrative Oncology for Clinicians and Cancer Patients: Part 4"
Townsend Letter. December 2011

"9 Things You Didn't Know About Detoxing"
Marie Claire. April 2015

"Pancreatic Cancer: Can Old Research Provide New Breakthroughs?"
USA Today. January 2014

"From an Ancient Peat, Nature's Powerful Cure"
Townsend Letter. November 2013

"Detoxification for Prostate Health"
Developing Health Habits / Men's Health. August 2011

"Use of Golden Leaf Ginkgo Extract for Skin Fibrosis"
Integrative Practitioner, 2010

"The Natural Approach to Cancer."
Townsend Letter. August & September. 2016, 64-67

"A Natural Approach to Cancer."
The American Chiropractor. November 11, 2016

ENDNOTES

Introduction

[1] Brawley, Otis. "The 40-Year War on Cancer." CNN. December 23, 2011. http://www.cnn.com/2011/12/23/health/forty-year-war/index.html.

[2] Hume, Tim, and Jen Christensen. "WHO: Cancer Cases to Rise 57% in 20 Years in 'Human Disaster.'" CNN. February 04, 2014. http://www.cnn.com/2014/02/04/health/who-world-cancer-report/index.html.

[3] Simon, Stacy. "Cancer Statistics Report: Death Rate Down 23% in 21 Years." American Cancer Society. January 7, 2016. https://www.cancer.org/latest-news/cancer-statistics-report-death-rate-down-23-percent-in-21-years.html.

[4] *Cancer Facts & Figures 2017*. Report. American Cancer Society. Atlanta, GA: 2017. 12. https://www.cancer.org/content/dam/cancer-org/research/cancer-facts-and-statistics/annual-cancer-facts-and-figures/2017/cancer-facts-and-figures-2017.pdf.

[5] Cuomo, Margaret I. *A World Without Cancer: The Making of a New Cure and the Real Promise of Prevention*. New York, NY: Rodale, 2013.

[6] Leaf, Clifton. "Why We're Losing the War on Cancer (And How to Win it)." *Fortune* 149, no. 6 (March 22, 2004).

[7] Buckland, Danny. "Will 2017 Be a Turning Point in the War Against Cancer?" Philips.

215

[8] Light, Donald W., and Hagop Kantarjian. "Market Spiral Pricing of Cancer Drugs." *Cancer* 119, no. 22 (September 03, 2013): 3900-902.

[9] Kantarjian, Hagop, David Steensma, Judit Rius Sanjuan, Adam Elshaug, and Donald Light. "High Cancer Drug Prices in the United States: Reasons and Proposed Solutions." *Journal of Oncology Practice* 10, no. 4 (July 2014): e208.

[10] Patterson, R. E., M. L. Neuhouser, M. M. Hedderson, S. M. Schwartz, L. J. Standish, and D. J. Bowen. "Changes in Diet, Physical Activity, and Supplement Use Among Adults Diagnosed with Cancer." *Journal of the American Dietetic Association* 103, no. 3 (March 2003): 323-28.

[11] Persistence Market Research. "Dietary Supplements Market is Expected to Reach US\$ 179.8 Billion, Globally in 2020: Persistence Market Research." News release, April 23, 2015. GlobeNewswire.

[12] Paller, Channing J., Samuel R. Denmeade, and Michael A. Carducci. "Challenges of Conducting Clinical Trials of Natural Products to Combat Cancer." *Clinical Advances in Hematology & Oncology* 14, no. 6 (June 2016): 448.

[13] Marty, M., J. M. Extra, M. Espie, S. Leandri, M. Besenval, and A. Krikorian. "Advances in Vinca-Alkaloids: Navelbine." *Nouvelle Revue Francaise D'hematologie* 31, no. 2 (January 1, 1989): 77-84.

[14] Cragg, G. M., and D. J. Newman. "Plants as a Source of Anti-Cancer Agents." *Journal of Ethnopharmacology* 100, no. 1-2 (August 22, 2005): 72-79.

Chapter 1

[1] "The Stem Cell Theory of Cancer." Ludwig Center for Cancer Stem Cell Research and Medicine. https://med.stanford.edu/ludwigcenter/overview/theory.html.

[2] Dr Gubler. Le Grand Secret. Plon. 1996.

[3] *Paris Match*. Vol. 2393. April 6, 1995.

[4] Denis Demonpion et Laurent Léger. Le dernier tabou, revelations sur la santé des Présidents. Pygmalion. 2012.

[5] Yu, Jun, Jeanne Drisko, and Qi Chen. "Inhibition of Pancreatic Cancer and Potentiation of Gemcitabine Effects by the Extract of Pao pereira." *Oncology Reports* 30, no. 1 (July 2013): 149-56.

[6] Yu, Jun, and Qi Chen. "The Plant Extract of Pao pereira Potentiates Carboplatin Effects Against Ovarian Cancer." *Pharmaceutical Biology* 52, no. 1 (January 2014): 36-43.

[7] Yu, Jun, and Qi Chen. "Antitumor Activities of Rauwolfia vomitoria Extract and Potentiation of Gemcitabine Effects Against Pancreatic Cancer." *Integrative Cancer Therapies* 13, no. 3 (May 2014): 217-25.

[8] Yu, Jun, Yan Ma, Jeanne Drisko, and Qi Chen. "Antitumor Activities of Rauwolfia vomitoria Extract and Potentiation of Carboplatin Effects Against Ovarian Cancer." *Current Therapeutic Research* 75 (December 2013): 8-14.

Chapter 2

[1] Monod, Jacques. Chance and Necessity: An Essay on the Natural Philosophy of Modern Biology. Knopf, 1971.

[2] Beljanski, Mirko. "Synthèse in vitro de l'ADN sur une matrice d'ARN par une transcriptase d'Escherichia coli." *Comptes Rendus de l'Académie des Sciences,* D, 274 (1972): 2801-804.

[3] Temin, Howard M. "Retrocitation." *Nature* 342, no. 6250 (December 7, 1989): 599-716.

[4] Shapiro, James A. "Revisiting the Central Dogma in the 21st Century." *Annals of the New York Academy of Sciences* 1178 (October 2009): 6.

[5] Malins, D. C., and S. J. Gunselman. "Fourier-transform Infrared Spectroscopy and Gas Chromatography-mass Spectrometry Reveal a Remarkable Degree of Structural Damage in the DNA of Wild Fish Exposed to Toxic Chemicals." *Proceedings of the National Academy of Sciences USA* 91, no. 26 (December 20, 1994): 13038-3041.

[6] Beljanski, Mirko. "Oncotest: a DNA Assay System for the Screening of Carcinogenic Substances." *IRCS Medical Science* 47 (1979): 218-25.

[7] Beljanski, Mirko, Liliane Le Goff, and Monique Beljanski. "In vitro Screening of Carcinogens Using DNA of the His-Mutant of Salmonella typhimurium." *Experimental Cell Biology* 50, no. 5 (1982): 271-80.

Chapter 3

[1] Chevret, Sophie. Enquête sur un survivant illégal. Paris: Guy Trédaniel Éditeur, 2002.

[2] Donadio, D., et al. "Tolerance and Feasibility of a 12-Month Therapy Using the Antiretroviral Agent PB100 in AIDS-Related Complex Patients." *Deutsche Zeitschrift für Onkologie* 26, no. 6 (1994).

[3] Brink, Anthony. "AZT: A Medicine from Hell." *Citizen*, March 17, 1999.

[4] Farber, Celia. "Sins of Omission: The Story of AZT, One of the Most Toxic, Expensive, and Controversial Drugs in the History of Medicine." *Spin* 5, no. 8, November 1989, 40.

[5] "AZT's Inhuman Cost." *The New York Times,* August 28, 1989.

[6] Marsa, Linda. "Toxic Hope: Widely Embraced, The Aids Drug Is Now Under Heavy Fire: The Azt Story." *Los Angeles Times,* June 20, 1993.

[7] Hookway, James. "Slumping Fertility Rates in Developing Countries Spark Labor Worries." *The Wall Street Journal* (New York), March 19, 2014.

[8] Guillette, Louis J., Jr., Daniel B. Pickford, D. Andrew Crain, Andrew A. Rooney, and H. Franklin Percival. "Reduction in Penis Size and Plasma Testosterone Concentrations in Juvenile Alligators Living in a Contaminated Environment." *General and Comparative Endocrinology* 101, no. 1 (January 1996): 32-42.

[9] Cavallini, Giorgio. "Environmental Pollution and Infertility." *Clinical Management of Male Infertility,* September 20, 2014, 165-71.

[10] Baker, Greg. "See You Later, Alligator Penis." *Miami New Times,* January 12, 1995.

Chapter 4

[1] Dr Gubler. Le Grand Secret. Plon. 1996.

[2] Okazaki, Reiji, Susumu Hirose, Tuneko Okazaki, Tohru Ogawa, and Yoshikazu Kurosawa. "Assay of RNA-Linked Nascent DNA Pieces with Polynucleotide Kinase." *Biochemical and Biophysical Research Communications* 62, no. 4 (February 1975): 1018-024.

[3] Beljanski, Mirko, and Michel Plawecki. "Particular RNA Fragments as Promoters of Leukocyte and Platelet Formation in Rabbits." *Experimental Cell Biology* 47, no. 3 (1979): 218-25.

[4] Beljanski, Mirko, Michel Plawecki, P. Bourgarel, and Monique Beljanski. "Short chain RNA Fragments as Promoters of Leucocyte and Platelet Genesis in Animals Depleted by Anti-Cancer Drugs." In the Role of RNA in Development and Reproduction. Sec. Int. Symposium. Science Press Beijing. M.C. Niu and H.H. Chuang Eds Van Nostrand Reinhold Company. (April 25-30, 1980): 79-113.

[5] Beljanski, Mirko. "The Regulation of DNA Replication and Transcription: The Role of Trigger Molecules in Normal and Malignant Gene Expression." *Experimental Biology and Medicine* 8 Karger (1983): 1-190.

[6] Beljanski, Mirko, and Michel Plawecki. "Particular RNA Fragments as Promoters of Leucocytes and Platelet Formations in Rabbits." *Experimental Cell Biology* 47 (1979): 218-25.

[7] Donadio, D., R. Lorho, J. E. Causse, T. Nawrocki, and Mirko Beljanski. "RNA Fragments (RLB) and Tolerance of Cytostatic Treatments in Hematology: A Preliminary Study about Two Non-Hodgkin Malignant Lymphoma Cases." *Deutsche Zeitschrift für Onkologie* 23, no. 2 (1991): 33-35.

[8] M. Beljanski. The anticancer agent PB-100, selectively active on malignant cells, inhibits multiplication of sixteen malignant cell lines, even multidrug resistant. *Genetics and Molecular Biology*, 23, 1, 29-33 (2000).

Chapter 5

[1] Nordau, Claudy G., and Monique Beljanski. *Beljanski: A Pioneer in Biomedicine: Concepts, Theories and Applications.* New York, NY: Edition EVI Liberty Corp., 2000.

[2] "Pills for Mental Illness?" *Time* 64, no. 19, November 8, 1954.

[3] Servier, Jacques. *Contribution à l'étude du Rauwolfia serpentina et aperçus sur quelques espèces voisines.* Master's thesis, Université Lille, 1957.

⁴ Stich, Rodney. *America's Medical Industry: The Good, the Bad, and the Deadly.* Alamo, CA: Silverpeak Publisher, Inc., 2012.

⁵ Hamdy, Ronald C. "Hypertension: A Turning Point in the History of Medicine...and Mankind." *Southern Medical Journal* 94, no. 11 (2001): 1045-047.

⁶ *Report on Carcinogens: Reserpine.* Report. National Toxicology Program. 14th ed. Research Triangle Park, NC: U.S. Department of Health and Human Services, Public Health Service, 2016. https://ntp.niehs.nih.gov/ntp/roc/content/profiles/reserpine.pdf.

⁷ Schoental, R. "Are Rauwolfia Alkaloids Carcinogenic?" *The Lancet* 304, no. 7896 (December 28, 1974): 1571.

⁸ Shapiro, S., J. L. Parsells, L. Rosenberg, D. W. Kaufman, P. D. Stolley, and D. Schottenfeld. "Risk of Breast Cancer in Relation to the use of Rauwolfia Alkaloids." *European Journal of Clinical Pharmacology* 26, no. 2 (1984): 143-46.

⁹ Stanford, Janet L., Elizabeth J. Martin, Louise A. Brinton, and Robert N. Hooever. "Rauwolfia Use and Breast Cancer: A Case-Control Study." *JNCI: Journal of the National Cancer Institute* 76, no. 5 (1986): 817-22.

¹⁰ Beljanski, Mirko, and Monique Beljanski. "Selective Inhibition of in vitro Synthesis of Cancer DNA by Alkaloids of β-Carboline Class." *Experimental Cell Biology* 50, no. 2 (1982): 79-87.

¹¹ Santos EC 1848. *Monografia do Geissospermum vellosii vulgo Pau-pereira.* Rio de Janeiro, 32p. These Inaugural, Faculdade de Medicina, Universidade Federal do Rio de Janeiro.

¹² M. Beljanski. The anticancer agent PB-100, selectively active on malignant cells, inhibits multiplication of sixteen malignant cell lines, even multidrug resistant. *Genetics and Molecular Biology*, 23, 1, 29-33 (2000).

Chapter 6

[1] *Sources and Effects of Ionizing Radiation*. Report. Scientific Committee on the Effects of Atomic Radiation, United Nations. Vol. 1. New York, NY: United Nations, 2000. 4.

[2] Bogo, V., C. G. Franz, A. J. Jacobs, J. F. Weiss, and R. W. Young. "Effects of Ehiofos (WR-2721) and Radiation on Monkey Visual Discrimination Performance." *Pharmacology & Therapeutics* 39, no. 1-3 (1988): 93-95.

[3] Kwant, Cor. "A-bombed Ginkgo Trees in Hiroshima, Japan." A-bombed Ginkgo Trees in Hiroshima, Japan. https://kwanten.home.xs4all.nl/hiroshima.htm.

[4] Causse, J. E., T. Nawrocki, and Mirko Beljanski. "Human Skin Fibrosis RNase Search for a Biological Inhibitor-Regulator." *Deutsche Zeitschrift für Onkologie* 26, no. 5 (1994): 137-39.

[5] Affaire Beljanski C. France-Arrêt Strasbourg 7 Février 2002 (Requête n° 44070/98).

[6] Schacter, Michael B. "Mirko Beljanski's Innovative Approach to Cancer, Chronic Viral Diseases and AutoImmune Conditions." *The Health Letter of FAIM The Foundation for the Advancement of Innovative Medicine,* Spring 2003.

[7] Davis, Devra. "Forward." In *The Regulation of DNA Replication and Transcription,* X, XV. 2nd ed. New York, NY: Demos Medical Publishing LLC, 2013.

[8] Beljanski, Mirko. "The Anticancer Agent PB-100, Selectively Active on Malignant Cells, Inhibits Multiplication of Sixteen Malignant Cell Lines, Even Multidrug Resistant." *Genetics and Molecular Biology* 23, no. 1 (2000): 29-33.

[9] Malins, D. C., and S. J. Gunselman. "Fourier-transform Infrared Spectroscopy and Gas Chromatography-mass Spectrometry Reveal a Remarkable Degree of Structural Damage in the DNA of Wild Fish Exposed to Toxic Chemicals." *Proceedings of the National Academy of Sciences USA* 91, no. 26 (December 20, 1994): 13038-3041.

Chapter 7

[1] "Key Statistics for Prostate Cancer." American Cancer Society. https://www.cancer.org/cancer/prostate-cancer/about/key-statistics.html.

[2] Beljanski, Mirko. "The Anticancer Agent PB-100, Selectively Active on Malignant cells, Inhibits Multiplication of Sixteen Malignant Cell Lines, Even Multidrug Resistant." *Genetics and Molecular Biology* 23, no. 1 (2000): 29-33.

[3] Bemis, Debra L., Jillian L. Capodice, Manisha Desai, Aaron E. Katz, and Ralph Buttyan. "β-Carboline Alkaloid-Enriched Extract from the Amazonian Rain Forest Tree Pao pereira Suppresses Prostate Cancer Cells." *Journal of the Society for Integrative Oncology* 7, no. 2 (Spring 2009): 59-65.

[4] D.L. Bemis, J.L. Capodice, P. Gorroochurn, A.E. Katz and R. Buttyan. Anti-prostate cancer activity of β-carboline alkaloid enriched extract from Rauwolfia vomitoria. *International Journal of Oncology,* 2006, 29: 1065-1073.

[5] Schachter, Michael B. "Integrative Oncology for Clinicians and Cancer Patients: Part 4." *Townsend Letter,* no. 341 (December 2011): 96.

[6] Coles, L. Stephen. *Extraordinary Healing: How the Discoveries of Mirko Beljanski, the World's First Green Molecular Biologist, Can Protect and Restore Your Health.* Topanga, CA: Freedom Press, 2011.

[7] Walker, Morton. *Cancer's Cause, Cancer's Cure: The Truth About Cancer, Its Causes, Cures, and Prevention.* Hugo House Publishers, Ltd., 2012.

[8] Hembery, R., A. Jenkins, G. White, and B. Richards. Illegal logging: Cut it out! *Report by World Wildlife Foundation* (WWF), UK.,2007.

[9] https://www.foe.co.uk/sites/default/files/downloads/import_illegal_timber.pdf http://www.fern.org/sites/fern.org/files/pubs/fw/srsep01.pdf

[10] Watts, Jonathan, and John Vidal. "Brazil Laundering Illegal Timber on a 'Massive and Growing Scale.'" *The Guardian.* May 14, 2014. https://www.theguardian.com/environment/2014/may/15/brazil-laundering-illegal-timber-on-a-massive-and-growing-scale.

[11] Huang, Suyun, Curtis A. Pettaway, Hisanori Uehara, Corazon D. Bucana, and Isaiah J. Fidler. "Blockade of NF-κB Activity in Human Prostate Cancer Cells is Associated with Suppression of Angiogenesis, Invasion, and Metastasis." *Oncogene* 20, no. 31 (July 12, 2001): 4188-197.

[12] Beljanski, Mirko, and S. Crochet. "The Selective Anticancer Agent PB-100 Inhibits Interleukin-6 Induced Enhancement of Glioblastoma Cell-Proliferation in-vitro." *International Journal of Oncology* 5 (October 1994): 873-79.

[13] Katz, Aaron E. "The Holistic Approach to Prostate Health." *Integrative Medicine* 6, no. 3 (June & July 2007).

Chapter 8

[1] Shapira, Michael Y., Pavel Kaspler, Simcha Samuel, Shmuel Shoshan, and Reuven Or. "Granulocyte Colony Stimulating Factor Does Not Induce Long-Term DNA Instability in Healthy Peripheral Blood Stem Cell Donors." *American Journal of Hematology* 73, no. 1 (May 2003): 33-36.

[2] Beljanski, Mirko. "Oncotest: A DNA Assay System for the Screening of Carcinogenic Substances." *IRCS Medical Science* 47 (1979): 218-25.

[3] Pulsipher, Michael A., Arnon Nagler, Robert Iannone, and Robert M. Nelson. "Weighing the Risks of G-CSF Administration, Leukopheresis, and Standard Marrow Harvest: Ethical and Safety Considerations for Normal Pediatric Hematopoietic Cell Donors." *Pediatric Blood & Cancer* 46, no. 4 (April 2006): 422-33.

[4] Pamphilon, D., E. Nacheva, C. Navarrete, A. Madrigal, and J. Goldman. "The Use of Granulocyte Colony-Stimulating Factor in Volunteer Blood and Marrow Registry Donors." *Bone Marrow Transplantation* 38, no. 10 (July 2006): 699-700.

[5] Anderlini, Paolo, and Richard E. Champlin. "Biologic and Molecular Effects of Granulocyte Colony-Stimulating Factor in Healthy Individuals: Recent Findings and Current Challenges." *Blood* 111, no. 4 (February 15, 2008): 1767-772.

[6] Anderlini, Paolo. "Effects and Safety of Granulocyte Colony-Stimulating Factor in Healthy Volunteers." *Current Opinion in Hematology* 16, no. 1 (January 2009): 35-40.

[7] Mccullough, Jeffrey, Jeffrey Kahn, John Adamson, Paolo Anderlini, Richard Benjamin, Dennis Confer, Mary Eapen, Betsy Hirsch, David Kuter, Ellen Lazarus, Derwood Pamphilon, David Stroncek, Jeremy Sugarman, and Robert Wilson. "Hematopoietic Growth Factors-Use in Normal Blood and Stem Cell Donors: Clinical and Ethical Issues." *Transfusion* 48, no. 9 (September 2008): 2008-025.

[8] Stephan, Pam. "What Is the Difference Between Neulasta and Neupogen?" Verywell. https://www.verywell.com/neulasta-vs-neupogen-for-chemotherapy-treatment-430223.

[9] Schiffer, Charles A., Kenneth C. Anderson, Charles L. Bennett, Steven Bernstein, Linda S. Elting, Miriam Goldsmith, Michael Goldstein, Heather Hume, Jeffrey J. McCullough, Rosemary E. McIntyre, Bayard L. Powell, John M. Rainey, Scott D. Rowley, Paolo Rebulla, Michael B. Troner, and Alton H. Wagnon. "Platelet Transfusion for Patients with Cancer: Clinical Practice Guidelines of the American Society of Clinical Oncology." *Journal of Clinical Oncology* 19, no. 5 (March 1, 2001): 1519-538.

[10] Elting, Linda S., Edward B. Rubenstein, Charles G. Martin, Danna Kurtin, Saul Rodriguez, Esa Laiho, Krishnakumari Kanesan, Scott B. Cantor, and Robert S. Benjamin. "Incidence, Cost, and Outcomes of Bleeding and Chemotherapy Dose Modification Among Solid Tumor Patients With Chemotherapy-Induced Thrombocytopenia." *Journal of Clinical Oncology* 19, no. 4 (February 15, 2001): 1137-146.

[11] Grimble, George K. "Why Are Dietary Nucleotides Essential Nutrients?" *British Journal of Nutrition* 76, no. 4 (October 1996): 475-78.

[12] Billioti de Gage, Sophie, Yola Moride, Thierry Ducruet, Tobias Kurth, Hélène Verdoux, Marie Tournier, Antoine Pariente, and Bernard Bégaud. "Benzodiazepine Use and Risk of Alzheimer's Disease: Case-Control Study." *BMJ* 349 (2014).

[13] Sloan, E. K., S. J. Priceman, B. F. Cox, S. Yu, M. A. Pimentel, V. Tangkanangnukul, J. M. G. Arevalo, K. Morizono, B. D. W. Karanikolas, L. Wu, A. K. Sood, and S. W. Cole. "The Sympathetic Nervous System Induces a Metastatic Switch in Primary Breast Cancer." *Cancer Research* 70, no. 18 (September 15, 2010): 7042-052.

[14] Carnegie, Dale. *How to Stop Worrying and Start Living.* Simon and Schuster, 1948.

[15] M. Beljanski. The Regulation of DNA Replication and Transcription. 3rd Edition Demos Medical Publishing-2013.

[16] Levin, Robert D., Maryann Daehler, James F. Grutsch, John L. Hall, Digant Gupta, and Christopher G. Lis. "Dose Escalation Study of an Anti-Thrombocytopenic Agent in Patients with Chemotherapy Induced Thrombocytopenia." *BMC Cancer* 10, no. 565 (October 19, 2010).

[17] "Important news for Chemotherapy and Radiotherapy Patients: If You Are Undergoing Chemotherapy or Radiotherapy, You Need to Know about ReaLBuild." *The Doctors' Prescription for Healthy Living,* November 2007, 24.

[18] Chang, Cunjie, Wei Zhao, Bingxian Xie, Yongming Deng, Tao Han, Yangyan Cui, Yundong Dai, Zhen Zhang, Jimin Gao, Hongqian Guo, and Jun Yan. "Pao pereira Extract Suppresses Castration-Resistant Prostate Cancer Cell Growth, Survival, and Invasion Through Inhibition of NFκB Signaling." *Integrative Cancer Therapies* 13, no. 3 (May 2014): 249-58.

[19] Walker, Morton. *Cancer's Cause, Cancer's Cure: The Truth About Cancer, Its Causes, Cures, and Prevention.* Hugo House Publishers, Ltd., 2012, 117-118.

[20] Burchill, Melissa. "Two Herbal Extracts for Protecting Prostate Cell DNA." *Integrative Medicine* 9, no. 2 (April & May 2010): 32-36.

[21] Coles, L. Stephen. "The Columbia Connection." *The Doctors' Prescription for Healthy Living* 14, no. 8, September 2010, 27.

[22] The MNT Editorial Team. "Pancreatic Cancer: Causes, Symptoms and Treatments." Medical News Today. January 05, 2016. https://www.medicalnewstoday.com/info/pancreatic-cancer.

Chapter 9

[1] Liu, Sa, S. Katharine Hammond, and Ann Rojas-Cheatham. "Concentrations and Potential Health Risks of Metals in Lip Products." *Environmental Health Perspectives* 121, no. 6 (June 2013): 705-10.

[2] Smallman, Etan. "From Arsenic in Rice to Toxic Metals in Sweets and Veg... Poisons in Your Shopping Basket." Daily Mail. November 17, 2014. http://www.dailymail.co.uk/femail/article-2836994/From-arsenic-rice-toxic-metals-sweets-veg-Poisons-shopping-basket.html.

[3] "Toxic Hepatitis." Mayo Clinic. October 04, 2016. http://www.mayoclinic.org/diseases-conditions/toxic-hepatitis/symptoms-causes/dxc-20251585.

[4] Beljanski, Mirko. "Oncotest: A DNA Assay System for the Screening of Carcinogenic Substances." *IRCS Medical Science* 47 (1979): 218-25.

[5] Robinson, Phil. "EDTA." *Chemistry World* (audio blog), April 4, 2012. https://www.chemistryworld.com/podcasts/edta/3005764.article.

[6] "Exclusive Interview with Garry Gordon, MD, DO: Oral Chelation for Improved Heart Function." *Life Enhancement,* April 1997.

[7] Goodman, Sara. "Tests Find More Than 200 Chemicals in Newborn Umbilical Cord Blood." Scientific American. December 2, 2009. https://www.scientificamerican.com/article/newborn-babies-chemicals-exposure-bpa/.

[8] BabyCenter Medical Advisory Board. "Are Plastic Baby Bottles Safe?" BabyCenter. June 20, 2016. https://www.babycenter.com/0_are-plastic-baby-bottles-safe_14387.bc.

[9] Cunningham, Vanessa. "10 Toxic Beauty Ingredients to Avoid." The Huffington Post. November 12, 2013. http://www.huffingtonpost.com/vanessa-cunningham/dangerous-beauty-products_b_4168587.html.

[10] Yu, Jun, and Qi Chen. "The Plant Extract of Pao pereira Potentiates Carboplatin Effects Against Ovarian Cancer." *Pharmaceutical Biology* 52, no. 1 (January 2014): 36-43.

[11] Yu, Jun, Yan Ma, Jeanne Drisko, and Qi Chen. "Antitumor Activities of Rauwolfia vomitoria Extract and Potentiation of Carboplatin Effects Against Ovarian Cancer." *Current Therapeutic Research* 75 (December 2013): 8-14.

[12] Yu, Jun, and Qi Chen. "Antitumor Activities of Rauwolfia vomitoria Extract and Potentiation of Gemcitabine Effects Against Pancreatic Cancer." *Integrative Cancer Therapies* 13, no. 3 (May 2014): 217-25.

[13] Yu, Jun, Jeanne Drisko, and Qi Chen. "Inhibition of Pancreatic Cancer and Potentiation of Gemcitabine Effects by the Extract of *Pao pereira.*" *Oncology Reports* 30, no. 1 (July 2013): 149-56.

[14] O'Brien, Dale. "Pancreatic Cancer Pre-Clinical Study (from an Amazonian Tree): Geissospermum vellosii." Pancreatica. August 20, 2013. http:// pancreatica.org/pre-clinical-study-of-natural-product-from-amazon-tree-geissospermum-vellosii/.

[15] Pert, Candace B. *Molecules of Emotion: The Science Behind Mind-Body Medicine.* New York, NY: Touchstone, 1999.

[16] "Phase 1 of Cancer: Inescapable Shock." Psycho-Oncology: Discover How Prolonged Chronic Stress Causes Cancer and How to Heal Within. http://www.alternative-cancer-care.com/.

[17] Sonnenburg, Justin, and Erica Sonnenburg. *The Good Gut: Taking Control of Your Weight, Your Mood, and Your Long-Term Health.* New York, NY: Penguin Books, 2016.

Chapter 10

1 *Commission pour les médicaments à base de plantes à usage humain.* Report. Agence fédérale des médicaments et des produits de santé. Brussels, Belgium, January 1, 2013. 1-4.

[2] Van Den Corput. *Le Journal de Médecine, de Chirurgie et de Phamacologie. Société Royale Des Sciences Medicales et Naturelles de Bruxelles.* Vol. 85. Brussels, Belgium: Librairie Medicale de H. Lamertin, 1887. 246.

[3] Puiseux, F., A. Le Hir, R. Goutarel, M. M. Janot, and J. Lemen. "On the Alkaloids of Pao-pereira, Geissospermum laeve (Vellozo) Baillon. Note III. Geissoschizoline, Apogeissoschizine and Geissospermine." *Annales Pharmaceutiques Francaises* 17 (Oct.-Dec. 1959): 626-33.

[4] Anderson, John W., and Larry Trivieri. *Alternative Medicine: The Definitive Guide.* 2nd ed. New York, NY: Celestial Arts, 2002.

[5] Lanctôt, Ghislaine. *The Medical Mafia: How to Get Out of It Alive and Take Back Our Health & Wealth.* 2002.

[6] Weeks, Bradford S. "FDA Admits Incompetence, People Dying - Sign Petition." WeeksMD. February 24, 2009.

[7] Scott, Dylan. "The Untold Story of TV's First Prescription Drug Ad." STAT, December 11, 2015. https://www.statnews.com/2015/12/11/untold-story-tvs-first-prescription-drug-ad/.

[8] Lo, Chris. "Big Pharma and the Ethics of TV Advertising." Pharmaceutical Technology. November 28, 2013. http://www.pharmaceutical-technology.com/features/feature-big-pharma-ethics-of-tv-advertising/.

[9] Steinman, David W. "Two Powerful Unique Herbs, Rauwolfia & Pao, Protect Prostate Cell DNA and Promote All Facets of Prostate Health." *The Doctors' Prescription for Healthy Living* 11, no. 12 (2008): 18-20.

[10] Leaf, Clifton. "Why We're Losing the War on Cancer (And How to Win it)." *Fortune* 149, no. 6 (March 22, 2004).

[11] Cagan, Michele. "Breakthrough Studies Reveal Miracle Plants Defeats the Two Most Incurable Cancer-Pancreatic and Ovarian." *Health Sciences Institute Members Alert* 18, No. 4 (December 2013).

[12] "Gemcitabine after Pancreatic Cancer Surgery Improves Survival." *National Cancer Institute Bulletin* 5, no. 12 (June 10, 2008): 1-2.

[13] Egnew, Thomas R. "Suffering, Meaning, and Healing: Challenges of Contemporary Medicine." *The Annals of Family Medicine* 7, no. 2 (March 2009): 170-75.

[14] Yu, Jun, Jeanne Drisko, and Qi Chen. "Inhibition of Pancreatic Cancer and Potentiation of Gemcitabine Effects by the Extract of Pao pereira." *Oncology Reports* 30, no. 1 (July 2013): 149-56.

[15] Yu, Jun, and Qi Chen. "Antitumor Activities of Rauwolfia vomitoria Extract and Potentiation of Gemcitabine Effects Against Pancreatic Cancer." *Integrative Cancer Therapies* 13, no. 3 (May 2014): 217-25.

[16] "Personalized Medicine 101: The Challenges." Personalized Medicine Coalition. http://pmc.blueonblue.com/Resources/Personalized_Medicine_101_The_Challenges.

Epilogue

[1] Beljanski, Mirko. "Synthèse in vitro de l'ADN sur une matrice d'ARN par une transcriptase d'Escherichia coli." *Comptes Rendus de l'Académie des Sciences* 274 (1972): 2801-804.

[2] Beljanski, Mirko, and Monique Beljanski. "RNA-Bound Reverse Transcriptase in Escherichia coli and in vitro Synthesis of a Complementary DNA." *Biochemical Genetics* 12 (1974): 163-80.

[3] Beljanski, Mirko, L. C. Niu, Monique Beljanski, S. Yan, and M. C. Niu. "Iron Stimulated RNA-Dependent DNA Polymerase Activity from Goldfish Eggs." *Cellular and Molecular Biology* 34 (1988): 17-25.